Springer
Berlin
Heidelberg
New York
Barcelona
Budapest
Hong Kong
London
Milan
Paris
Santa Clara
Singapore
Tokyo

Ross Anderson (Ed.)

Personal Medical Information

Security, Engineering, and Ethics

Personal Information Workshop
Cambridge, UK, June 21-22, 1996
Proceedings

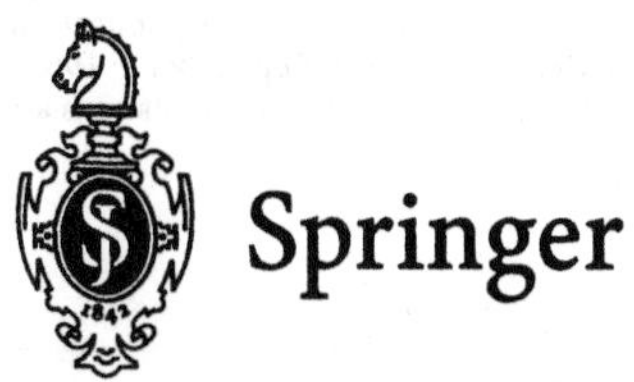

Volume Editor

Ross Anderson
University of Cambridge, Computer Laboratory
New Museums Site, Pembroke Street, Cambridge CB2 3QG, UK
E-mail: rja14@cl.cam.ac.uk

Cataloging-in-Publication data applied for

Die Deutsche Bibliothek - CIP-Einheitsaufnahme

Personal medical information : security, engineering, and ethics ; personal information workshop, Cambridge, UK, June 21 - 22, 1996 ; proceedings / Ross Anderson (ed.). - Berlin ; Heidelberg ; New York ; Barcelona ; Budapest ; Hong Kong ; London ; Milan ; Paris ; Santa Clara ; Singapore ; Tokyo : Springer, 1997
ISBN 3-540-63244-1

CR Subject Classification (1991): K.6.5, E.3, J.3, H.2.0

ISBN 3-540-63244-1 Springer-Verlag Berlin Heidelberg New York

Typesetting: Camera-ready by author
SPIN 10634364 06/3142 – 5 4 3 2 1 0 Printed on acid-free paper

Foreword

In the last few years, the protection of computerised medical records, and of other personal health information, has become the subject of both technical research and political dispute in a number of countries.

In Britain, the issue arose initially as an argument between the British Medical Association and the Department of Health over whether encryption should be used in a new medical network. In Germany, the focus was the issue to all patients of a smartcard to hold insurance details and facilitate payment; while in the USA, the debate has been whether federal law should preempt state regulation of computerised medical records, and if so, what technical and legal protection should be afforded the patient.

Whatever the origin and evolution of this debate in specific countries, it has become clear that policy and technical matters are closely intertwined. What does 'computer security' mean in the medical context? What are we trying to do? What are the threats that we are trying to forestall? What costs might reasonably be incurred? To what extent is the existing technology — largely developed to meet military and banking requirements — of use? And perhaps hardest of all, what is the right balance between technical and legal controls?

As the debate spread, it became clear that there was little serious contact between the people who could state the requirements — clinical professionals, medical ethicists and patients — and the people who could explore how to meet these requirements, most (but not all) of them from the computer security community. How could this gap be bridged?

It so happened that from January to June 1996, I was organising a six-month research programme in computer security, cryptology, and coding theory at the Isaac Newton Institute for Mathematical Sciences in Cambridge. This would be attended by most of the top researchers in the field, and seemed too good an opportunity to miss. I brought it to the attention of the BMA, and it was agreed that the Isaac Newton Institute and the BMA would jointly sponsor a two-day interdisciplinary workshop focussed on medical computer security and entitled *'Personal Information — Security, Engineering and Ethics'*.

The conference was opened by the President of the BMA, Sir Terence English, and the first item of business was the announcement of an agreement between the BMA and UK health data processing companies on standards for the de-identification of personal health information kept for such purposes as computing hospital readmission rates and referral patterns. The papers presented here were then delivered, and for the following two days we had a lively exchange of views between doctors, lawyers, privacy activists, medical informatics professionals, and the computer security community.

The papers in these proceedings reflect this breadth of interest. The origin of the debate between the BMA and the British government are described in the papers by Simon Jenkins and Fleur Fisher, while its history is set out in the paper by Ross Anderson who also describes the BMA's approach to safety and privacy that developed out of it. A pilot project to implement the BMA's recommendations is reported on by Alan Hassey and Mike Wells. Alternative views are presented by Ruth Roberts, Joyce Thomas, Mike Rigby, John Williams, and Andrew Blyth. Mary Hawking sets out the viewpoint of a primary care physician, while Peter Landrock and John Williams describe a prototype system for securing clinical messages between primary carers and the hospital.

Four German papers were given. Anja Hartmann and Otto Ulrich present the viewpoint of the BSI (the German government's information security agency); Bernd Blobel discusses the measures taken to bring the former East German cancer registries up to Western standards of privacy protection after the fall of the Berlin Wall; Ulrich Kohl describes an access control system built for a German hospital; while Gerrit Bleumer and Matthias Schunter show how cryptographic mechanisms can provide ways to clear healthcare payments so that patients remain anonymous while insurers can still control costs.

Compared with Britain and Germany, the US concerns are more at the policy level, and concern how the interests of insurers and patients can be reconciled by legislative mechanisms (absent the kind of system described by Bleumer and Schunter). The privacy activists' position is stated by Beverly Woodward; Reid Cushman asks why healthcare systems are at all special; and the practical problems are elucidated by Agneta Breitenstein. Having heard of the situation in the USA, delegates endorsed the motion that: *"This meeting deplores the disaster in medical privacy threatened in the USA by proposals to legitimise the widespread sharing of personal health information without patient consent; and would also deplore similar developments in Europe and elsewhere."*

The remaining three papers each come from different countries. Ronald Draper discusses how an Irish hospital's systems deal with the privacy of mental health information; a Japanese health smartcard project is described by Yoshikazu Okada, Yasuo Haruki, Youichi Ogushi, and Masanobu Horie; while finally Roddy Neame describes the healthcare system in New Zealand. This appears to meet many of the privacy requirements and aspirations of other countries, with the data kept centrally for research and audit purposes being de-identified.

Taken together, the papers in this volume give a snapshot not merely of the state of the medical computer security art at the middle of 1996, but of the complex interplay between the technical, political, and human aspects of medical informatics which make it so fascinating.

We hope that this volume of proceedings will contribute to the development of policies and mechanisms to protect the safety and privacy of clinical information, and to establishing clinical information security as a distinct engineering discipline. The ultimate goal is that both patients and healthcare professionals should derive the greatest possible benefit from information technology; and we are grateful to the BMA and the Isaac Newton Institute for enabling us to take a few small but important steps in this direction.

Ross Anderson
January 1997

PERSONAL INFORMATION

Security, Engineering and Ethics

Cambridge, England
June 21–22, 1996

Sponsored by the

Isaac Newton Institute for Mathematical Sciences

and the

British Medical Association

Chair

Ross Anderson, University of Cambridge, UK

Programme Committee

Ab Bakker .... Bazis, The Netherlands
David Banisar .... Electronic Privacy Information Center, USA
Gerrit Bleumer .... University of Hildesheim, Germany
Paula Bruening .... Formerly Office of Technology Assessment, USA
Ian Cheong .... RACGP, Australia
Fleur Fisher .... British Medical Association, UK
Elizabeth France .... Data Protection Registrar, UK
Bob Frankford .... Formerly Ontario Legislature, Canada
Peter Landrock .... Århus University, Denmark
Robert Morris .... NSA, USA
Roderick Neame .... Health Information Consulting, UK
Roger Needham .... University of Cambridge, UK
Beverly Woodward .... Brandeis University, USA

Contents

Information and the NHS
(For me or for them?)

Simon Jenkins MBE FRCGP

General Practitioner, The Minden Medical Centre, Bury
Chairman of BMA's Information Technology Committee

21 June 1996

Before discussing the Information and Technology strategy of the NHS, we must consider the objectives of that strategy and whether they are legitimate.

Government objectives are to provide for and protect the health of the public they serve. They must ensure that all citizens have access to necessary care, free at the time of need; they must ensure that the public health is maintained and improved; and they must provide the necessary finance to fund these objectives primarily out of general taxation. (These principles are set out in parliamentary language in the various NHS Acts, since 1946).

These objectives generate a central government imperative to "control expenditure", and to get the best possible "value for money". They imply a mechanism for monitoring expenditure; for measuring what is being provided; for identifying gaps in provision, and for closing those gaps.

There are further considerations that derive from these objectives and apply to any area of public spending. For example:

1. How efficient, effective and equitable are the resource distribution, control and monitoring mechanisms?
2. Can fraud be detected?
3. Is money being spent effectively or wasted, and how is it being wasted?
4. Is the service responsive to the changing (health care) needs of the population?
5. Are the bureaucratic mechanisms consuming more of the (health care) resources than they should, and how can excessive bureaucracy be reduced?

These questions are posed from the legitimate prospective of government. The other quite different but equally legitimate approach is to ask what individual patients want from the people who provide their healthcare services. The patients perspective is by its very nature different from that of government.

The medical profession (and the BMA) must ask is which set of principles should doctors follow in providing their services to individual patients and the community.

These can be considered as follows:

Principle One: Standards - "Best Possible Care"

> *Doctors must provide the best possible care to the individual patient who consults them within the resources (time, facilities, and funding available), referring to other health care providers where appropriate.*

Principle Two: Confidentiality

> *In pursuing the first principle, doctors must ensure the confidentiality of the consultation is protected, subject to clearly defined exceptions which must be clarified by legislation (see draft bill on Disclosure of Personal Health Information - The Lord Walton Bill[1]). To ensure that the confidentiality of information given in consultations is maintained, they should adhere to the nine principles set out in the BMA Security Policy[2] commissioned from Dr Ross Anderson, which are derived from the GMC's Guidance "Good Medical Practice"[3].*

Principle Three: Public health advice

> *Doctors must advise on matters of "public health" that relate to their communities or to larger groups of the population.*
>
> *Doctors and other healthcare professionals may act as policy makers in their own right or may advise others who are responsible for determining the resources, nature and range of healthcare services.*

The role of the doctor as a provider of medical advice and treatment to individuals must not be confused with the separate and arguably equally important role as an advisor to healthcare organisations. The cash limiting of resources for healthcare will inevitably force a conflict of interest between these two roles.

Compromise solutions must be arrived at through honest and open debate between those who advocate and those who allocate on behalf of patients.

A single doctor can carry out both functions but it should be clear to all when he or she is acting as advocate or allocator and for whom they are acting at any given time. Lack of clarity leads to mistrust by individual patients or accusations by healthcare organisations that the doctor has a vested interest and cannot give unbiased advice.

Education, teaching and research are other aspects of the responsibilities of doctors referred to in the GMC's Guidance on "Good Medical Practice", but it is the first three principles enunciated above that are the rock upon which ethical medical practice can flourish in a system of healthcare provision where a third party (ie. neither the doctor nor the patient) have accepted responsibility for paying for the consultation and the interventions that flow from it, which together form the health services.

There is a view that where a third party is paying for health care, that third party has a right to know what they are paying for, and whether it represents value for money.

If the patient is paying directly for the medical services then there is no conflict.

However, if an Insurance Company is paying, the Insurance Company must balance their payments for treatment of those clients who are sick against the interests of maintaining lower premiums for the totality of their clientele. The company will take appropriate action either to maintain profit margins, or in the case of a non-profit organisation, to maintain its membership levels.

The same imperatives will apply to a government in a National Health System, and by logical implication to its purchasing subsidiaries.

The crucial questions that set the scene for a conflict of interests are:

1. How much detail do paying authorities need to know to carry out their legitimate functions?
2. Do individual patients have to "consent" to their personal details being made known to "others" for the benefit of the organisation itself, and if so to what extent?
3. What is the precise point of conflict between the needs of the organisation or institution, and the personal privacy of individual patients?

The BMA has adopted a twin track approach to finding a solution which lies at the heart of this conflict.

Firstly, the draft Bill on Disclosure of Personal Health Information (The Lord Walton Bill) will ensure that the rules for breaching confidentiality are explicit and enshrined in legislation, and the penalties for breach of confidentiality can be made clear to all.

Secondly, the BMA Security Policy will encourage all involved in health care provision to use procedures and record systems that uphold the GMC rules for good medical practice.

We can all be accused from time to time of sloppy practices over how we have "secured" our written medical records, but they can be no excuse for basing developments in medical recording on what are already known to be bad standards of practice. To rely on illegibility as a means of keeping recorded information confidential, is a damming recognition of the inherent inadequacy and vulnerability of paper records to unauthorised access. But, when laissez-faire practices surrounding written records are transferred to new media, previously unknown but even greater dangers may arise. Uncontrolled, unauthorised, and undetected access to view let alone alter a record threatens the fundamental requirements of patient consent and confidentiality. The power of medical record aggregation is another new threat to individual liberties.

The future challenge lies not only in harnessing the advantages that technology can bring but in addressing the deficiencies of past and present styles of practice.

An outstanding matter for resolution is to determine what level of consent is adequate to protect the interests of an individual who is the subject of care, from the interests of the institution or organisation who provides that care. Is it sufficient for consent to be assumed to have been given if a patient presents him or herself for treatment? Such "implied consent", if it is used, can only be implied for immediate clinical care and not for any other organisational activity that takes place outside the consultation. It is most certainly not appropriate to assume such consent has been given for "potential" patients who have not yet presented themselves for treatment.

Only full and informed consent, freely given by an individual can guarantee the privacy of that individual. An institution that upholds this principle will acquire a reputation of respect, trust, and fairness which will enhance the confidence not only of those who work in it, but also those who call upon it for services.

The rights and responsibilities of patients and providers will become clearer, in a system that ensures that when a conflict of interest does occur it is resolved openly and the grounds for making the judgement are subject to public scrutiny.

Expensive, bureaucratic control mechanisms do not promote trust, either by the patients in the institution itself, or by those who work for it. If the institution trusts those who provide its services, and if patients acquire a sense of ownership of and responsibility towards the institution, better value for money will result. Those who provide services will be motivated to ensure that their services are of high quality, efficient, and effective and those who use them will do so responsibly, carefully, and without abuse.

Pitfalls along the road of change

We can list the steps along the road of change in the administration of the NHS which have diminished patients' self reliance and their sense of personal responsibility for the National Health Service. These trends have been encouraged and accelerated by the decisions of those driving and controlling the organisational changes.

Leaving aside a decline in the uncritical acceptance of imposed authoritarianism and the erosion of many traditional social and moral values which inevitably affect all citizens and public institutions, I will discuss only the specific events and decisions that have posed threats to confidentiality within the NHS, particularly the failure to obtain explicit consent from those people who avail themselves of its services.

1. "Consent", "need to know", and the data protection act

In the late 1970's discussions in parliament and society in general were coming to a head regarding a need to protect data in the new environment of computerisation that was starting to emerge[4]. This was of particular concern to the BMA and other health care professions, and as a result the Inter-Professional Working Group (IPWG) on Data Protection was established in 1981, chaired by Sir Douglas Black[5]. The main reason for setting up this group was the prediction that health authorities would be recognised as the "data users" under the proposed Data Protection Act. It would therefore be a health authority that would determine what happened to the information collected and recorded by the doctors, nurses and other health care professionals they employed, rather than the health care professionals themselves.

The difficult questions of how to define "consent" and "the rules that should govern the disclosure of information without consent", had to be faced. For many years the Department of Health evaded answering these questions. Indeed, they resisted publishing the "Code of Confidentiality" and its accompanying explanatory handbook which had been completed as the result of 60 meetings of the IPWG, and was available for publication in 1986. The Data Protection Act of 1984 was implemented in stages. The Subject Access Provisions of the Data Protection Act came into effect in 1987, which meant that a Health Authority having been recognised under the Act as the data user, could hold information about a patient and disclose it at will, and in certain circumstances could prevent the subject from having access to that information on the grounds that it may either cause that individual serious physical or mental harm, or could identify a third party who had provided some of the information, as long as that third party was not a health care professional.

Because these vital questions were not resolved, the matter grumbled on and is responsible for our present conflict with the Department of Health. Although the Department has gradually moved towards the views expressed by the IPWG, its progress has been painfully slow and their relative intransigence has consumed an enormous amount of valuable professional time. Although Government did not give support to the Lord Walton Bill this year at its first and second readings in the House of Lords, when it has to comply with the forthcoming European Legislation it may have to take onboard many of the matters raised by the Lord Walton Bill. (This Bill was derived from the original Inter-Professional Working Group's Code of Confidentiality formulated many years ago).

To date, the Department have consistently failed to produce adequate guidance on "informed consent" and "need to know". If they were to endorse the principles enunciated in the BMA's document on Security in Clinical Information Systems, it would go a long way to resolve matters. We could then jointly work out how current administrative and professional practices should change, such that the NHS will be seen to adopt "informed consent" and "the confidentiality of the consultation" as its fundamental ethos.

It is fortunate that in 1987 general practitioners negotiated with the Data Protection Registrar an agreement that permitted GP partnerships to be registered under the Data Protection Act as "data users"[6]. This enabled the patients of GP practices to be better protected than those who attended health authorities or community units for their care. The difference lay in the fact that the GP was both clinician and the person in control of the administration and management of the practice. It was the GP's registration as a doctor with the General Medical Council that ensured an extra level of protection of patients' data, over and above that provided by the Data Protection Act itself, in so far as GP's, like all other doctors, had to comply with their ethical principles. They therefore had a "legal" obligation to guarantee that their consultations were confidential, and that they obtained informed consent regarding disclosures.

Furthermore, their responsibilities extended beyond the strictures of the Data Protection Act and covered all communications, whether spoken, written, or transmitted by electronic means.

2. The screening obligations of health authorities and patients' consent

As a result of the unfortunate death of a patient from cervical cancer due to a failure of the administrative system for cervical cytology follow-up, Kenneth Clarke as Secretary of State for Health, placed an obligation on health authorities to implement a failsafe system of follow-up. To achieve this laudable objective, health authorities were obliged to gain access to FHSA registers. The FHSA registers held information from GP's about the cervical smear claims that they had submitted. At that time patients signed consent forms for each cervical smear test that was carried out, and thus gave permission for the general practitioners to submit a claim for item of service payment. In so doing patients "authorised" their data to be sent to the FHSA for that purpose.

As a result of the Kenneth Clarke action, all smears taken by any agency in any location became part of the register. The recall system, for those patients who had previously had cervical smears, was located in FHSA's but their population registers were then also used to identify and contact patients who had never had a smear. It was the responsibility of the Director of Public Health to ensure adequate follow-up mechanisms were in place and any abnormal smears were pursued. One of the failsafe mechanisms required the consultant in charge of the cervical cytology laboratory to set up another record system to make sure that any abnormal smears discovered by the laboratory were chased up. The operation of the recall system, which was the responsibility of the health authority, was devolved to the FHSA. The FHSA register was thus, by default, outside "clinical control". Additional clinical information such as whether the patient had had a hysterectomy for non-malignant disease, and therefore no longer needed to be recalled for a cervical smear was sent to the Register by GP's or by health authorities without the informed consent of patients. The fact that a patient was being followed up at a local hospital because of an abnormal smear was also notified to the FHSA Register, again without the patient's consent.

The introduction of targets for cervical cytology into the GP Contract in 1990 encouraged GP's to give more accurate information about hysterectomised women to FHSA's. Individual women are not asked to consent to this changed procedure. There should be a mechanism to ensure that such consent is sought in future.

The unquestionable value of a comprehensive programme for cervical cancer screening to individual women should not be allowed to over-ride their right to consent to be involved in the programme, or indeed not to be involved. They should also be made aware of the information given to FHSA's by various agencies, and of the security measures that surround the data bases. They should also be made aware of the identity of the people who access the registers.

3. Compulsory sharing of authority data by political decree rather then by public debate

Sharing of data between previously "independent" FHSA's and their associated District Health Authorities was achieved without public debate and without asking the consent of those individuals to whom these data related.

Since the inception of the NHS, the Executive Councils, FPC's, and subsequently FHSA's had all regarded data about patients and general practitioners as highly confidential, and had jealously guarded their data bases with a high standard of security. Their patient registers were held, originally in manual form and only later became computerised. Authority members of an FHSA were debarred from access to the register, even though some may have wished to know how many patients were registered with a particular doctor, or whether a particular patient was registered with a particular doctor. They were debarred from having this information on grounds of confidentiality and their status as an FHSA member did not confer an automatic right to the data held by their "authority". This attitude to security could occasionally be perceived as an obstruction to providing care. For example, when a patient changed their GP and the former GP wished to pass on some important clinical information, the FHSA would not reveal the name and address of the new doctor, although they would forward the necessary information in a sealed envelope to the new doctor.

Health Authorities were often irritated, particularly nurse managers of community nursing personnel, because if they knew the age/sex structure of a particular practice, they would be better able to allocate their nursing staff to the primary care team of that practice, instead of having to rely solely on advice from the practice about its need for additional attached staff.

Because of such perceived impediments to the planning requirements of health authorities, and also in anticipation of the NHS reforms, there was a government imperative to ensure that FHSA's and health authorities should share their data. This was a clear example of the needs of the organisation overriding the interests of individual patients and healthcare professionals for the deemed benefit of the population as a whole. The BMA resisted this action. The GMSC pressed for a parliamentary debate on the matter of compulsory data sharing by different health authorities. In retrospect the profession should have pressed for a public rather than a parliamentary debate. However, there was no true parliamentary debate, merely a statement by the Minister of Health (Mr Roger Freeman) during a committee stage of the NHS Bill[7]. His 30 second statement declared that "in future FHSA's will share their data with health authorities".

His argument was that this was needed for the "provision of seamless care", and our objections were to no avail. Seamless care has the connotation of being clinically required, but all the actions that flow from signing up to this philosophy are administratively driven. Whilst seamless care is necessary to ensure that patients obtain the most appropriate care in the most appropriate place, by the most appropriate health care professional, in fact seamless care is a means of ensuring that administrative procedures are carried out by more centralised authorities, rather than duplicated by smaller peripheral ones. Multiple small administrative mistakes are thus less likely, but the opportunity for single greater errors and dangers with greater impact is enhanced.

4. Clinical or administrative determinants in reimbursement policies – The effects on GP computing

It is unnecessary if general practitioners have set up call and recall procedures for patients who are registered with their practices, to duplicate the exercise by similar call and recall mechanisms at the FHSA level. If health authorities trust general practitioners to provide a screening service, then it should be unnecessary for an administrative failsafe mechanism also to be set up, unless the reason is to protect the Secretary of State and the health authorities from litigation or embarrassment. The prime purpose of any programme should be to improve the uptake of smear testing, and the follow-up of abnormal smears in the population. General practitioners are far more effective in persuading patients to have the procedures carried out than other agencies. High response rates for any screening or immunisation programme are better when organised by GPs because when patients are contacted by their general practitioner, with whom they have an existing relationship and whom they trust, they are more likely to respond to positively[8]. Furthermore, UK general practice, with stable lists of registered patients who consult the GP for a wide range of reasons, provides the ideal environment for opportunistic screening of defaulting responders. If health authorities are concerned about unregistered patients, they should encourage them to register with a general practitioner. To offer the screening service directly to this group of patients will take up such a disproportionate effort and resource that it will not be cost effective.

The government recognised the effectiveness of general practitioners to implement public health measures when, with the 1990 GP contract, target payments for cervical cytology and immunisation were introduced. They also acknowledged that the practice based computer was an essential tool for this exercise and allowed 50% of the purchase and running costs of GP computers to be reimbursed. Before that time, GP's were responsible for the whole cost of their practice computing activities and as a result developments in GP computing were clinically driven and geared towards solving practice based problems. The management of repeat prescribing which was a major burden on practices in the United Kingdom was an area in which patient care could be demonstrably improved by its proper control. At that time GP's and their computer suppliers were not distracted by the requirements of the administration. They directed their energies towards solving "GP perceived" problems.

There was also a "research ethic" which was a spin-off of the high level of morale that existed in general practice in the early 1980's. It was deemed important to develop age-sex morbidity registers at practice level so that patients with chronic disease could be managed proactively. Patients who were registered but did not attend the doctor could be identified and screened for problems where early intervention may bring benefit. The example par excellence was the identification of patients with previously unreported coronary risk factors[9].

Many of these ideas were promoted by the profession in a way that practices found acceptable. However, when they were embodied in the 1990 Contract, to become the norm for all practices, a penal attitude was introduced towards those who did not reach the imposed target level. Those who did achieve the targets were rewarded with payments, which were regarded as being removed from their colleagues who were less successful. There was insufficient recognition that the priorities of patients and practices in one area may be different from the national norm. The oppressive nature of perceived contractual financial penalties diverted attention away from individual practices identifying and finding solutions to their own particular local needs.

As long as the reimbursement for GP computing was based principally on the practice's own decisions about priorities, developments in GP computing were underpinned by the clinical needs of practices. But when the major element of reimbursement was determined by the management needs of the FHSA or health authority, the clinically driven pressure for development in GP computing was diminished. The 100% reimbursement of the capital costs of GP Fundholding and 75% of their running costs was a clear example of the diversion of development effort. If, as is expected, GP Links are reimbursed by health authorities at 100%, it will encourage GP computer suppliers to respond to the priorities of FHSA's and health authorities rather than those of practices. Developments in GP computing will become increasingly less clinically led and the interests of the organisation will be favoured over those that support practice based services to patients.

5. Contracting, confidentiality, and GP computing

The internal market in the NHS is founded on contracts between purchases and providers, and a major driver of that process has been the creation of GP fundholding. As a consequence a new range of requirements for GP computing was spawned. The emphasis related principally to the secondary care needs of registered patients, rather than the primary care demands of the patients as they present to general practitioners and their primary health care teams.

In 1989/1990 I commented at length on the first specification of GP Fundholding software[10]. I concluded that it did not address the problems that needed to be solved in general practice; it related solely to secondary care and it would be a burden to general practitioners. The very fact that 100% of the hardware costs and 75% of the software was to be reimbursed, underlined government determination to place GP Fundholding in the vanguard of establishing the internal market in the NHS, with the expectation that GP purchasing would control secondary care costs.

There were many casualties in this process, in particular confidentiality but also the time available for dealing with the problems that patients presented to their general practitioners was reduced, as more professional time was diverted to monitoring the secondary care activity of the patients they had referred to specialists.

Health authorities became more involved with the health of their communities, rather than focusing their main attention on secondary care. They tried to identify patients with problems before they presented symptomatically in an attempt to reduce the burden of acute serious illness. Some community units sought to develop their own empires in primary care, believing that they could be more effective than GP based primary health care teams.

In 1981[11], I suggested that screening programmes should be embedded in general practice and not divorced from it. If health authorities create separate administrative structures for each condition to be screened, the result will be excessively bureaucratic, less effective, and for more expensive in terms of the demands on medical and nursing manpower.

By embedding clinical information in contracting, without the constraints placed upon clinicians by their ethical codes of practice, and the adoption of administrative programmes of selective screening without the involvement of the protective buffer of general practice, far more information about individual patients has been placed in the hands of NHS employees who would not normally have regular contact with those patients, and certainly not their informed consent to use it and control it.

6. The rights of the "NHS family" versus the privacy of individual patients

The shared Electronic Patient Record for acute hospitals is a major project flowing from the IM&T Strategy. The questions of how informed consent has been sought and whether adequate safeguards for the security and confidentiality of personal health data have been addressed in this major IMG project, need to be thoroughly examined. However, sharing is part of its philosophy.

The government's view of the NHS family was that personal health information should be widely available on a need to know basis, in order to provide adequate care. I criticised this attitude in 1991[12] on the grounds that it was cavalier. The presumption was that any non-clinical manager who decided on a set of unpublished and often "self-determined" rules, that he had a need to know, could access the patient record without asking the patient's permission, since that permission would have been deemed implicitly given by the patient when they were seen in hospital. At that time it was suggested that the general practitioner's record should be similarly accessible if there was a need to know. Thankfully this latter view is no longer fashionable.

In all the IM&T Infrastructure projects there has been a proviso that confidentiality must be upheld, but this proviso has never prevented a project from proceeding, partly because no satisfactory definition of confidentiality and need to know has been reached. It is only when embarrassing breaches of confidentiality occur, such as incidents that led to the creation of "Safe Havens" in health authorities and Trusts, that political and subsequent administrative action has been taken to counter breaches[13]. The BMA's "Security Policy for Clinical Information Systems" is the mechanism whereby "confidentiality" can now be placed at the top of the list in any proposal and will form the basis for projects to demonstrate how "consent" and "need to know" can be unequivocally defined and practically implemented. Only when this approach is adopted with vigour and sincerity will all the anticipated benefits that can flow from the use of electronic records and communication be achieved.

Solving the problem of confidentiality and security in the shared Electronic Patient Record project is clearly a major task for hospital clinicians, but it is also increasingly relevant in terms of defining access, authorization, audit trails, consent, and need to know, for large group practices with more and more health professionals involved in primary health care teams.

7. From whom shall data be collected?

General practitioner records are complex structures. The principles underlying this complexity have been teased out by Rector, Nolan and Kay[14].

Any agency that attempts to derive data from such records should be aware of this seminal publication.

Their first assumption was that "the principle purpose of the medical record is to support individual patient care".

Their second assumption was that all clinical information will be held in a structured representation that can be manipulated by the system. What is recorded is what is observed and believed by the clinician, and not necessarily what is "true" about the patient.

The implications for extracting data for other purposes when these assumptions are understood are considerable. Amalgamated data from this source will represent an extract of clinical observations and opinions rather than what is necessarily true of the events that were observed. If one wishes to undertake research or collect epidemiological information, then the systems that are designed for this purpose will be different from those designed to support individual patient care. A good clinical medical record for individual patient care will facilitate descriptive recording, whereas for research and epidemiological purposes it will be prescriptive in nature, and indicate what information needs to be collected for the stated objectives of the research or epidemiology.

Leaving aside these fundamental considerations, there are a number of other important matters raised by the desire to collect data from health care professionals.

The Arthur Anderson report[15] that looked at the Administration of the Family Practitioner Services in the 1970's, and Mrs. Korner in her many reports in the 1980's on the information requirements of the NHS[16], both expressed views about the collection of data by health care professionals. They believed that:-

a) "Data should be collected once and once only.
b) Any management data should be derived from operational data.
c) Such data should be fed back to those who collected it in order to determine whether it represented the reality of the clinical interface.

d) Any data for management should not be an additional burden on those who had to collect it."

Despite such received wisdom, management has rarely taken notice of these exhortations.

Furthermore it is surprising, despite the enormous effort that has gone into defining minimum data sets, how scant consideration has been given by management to the precise and minimal information that they require at different levels within the organisation to make decisions relevant to their functions of allocation of resources, and monitoring the volume and quality of services that are delivered.

Great emphasis is placed on identifying the components of a process that can be counted and manipulated. For example, patients and staff can be counted, waiting times or lists can be measured, "completed consultant episodes" can be determined; and in the contracting environment of the internal market the volume, type, and cost of the transactions can be amalgamated into firm figures, in the certain knowledge that they have been derived from actual contractual activity.

Inevitably, the less easily countable or defined elements of service provision such as quality, compassion, and kindness - all of which may consume costly time are "devalued" when judging the overall cost/benefit of service measurements where one half of the equation is more sharply quantified. The information that is "missing" or "not quantifiable", can be called "soft" information. Managers may state that such "soft" information is used to put the hard data into context, and indeed to interpret it, but not infrequently those who provide the "soft" information (a euphemism for professional advice) have difficulty in understanding the reasoning behind the measurements that have been made, and have their work cut out to prevent action being taken on the hard data alone. All too rarely in the NHS management structure is "soft" information - (or professional advice) - the driving force for collecting data that will support or refute management strategy. Increasingly, management decisions have been made on the basis of political ideology, such that data is sought to support preconceived opinions. The accepted scientific approach is to formulate an hypothesis, and then seek to disprove it. Such critical appraisal leads to many practical failures, but moves knowledge and understanding progressively nearer to the truth.

The data needs at each level of decision making must therefore be carefully and critically evaluated before instructions for data collection are propagated.

When FHSA's were asked in the late 80's and early 90's to assess the health needs of their populations, there was a rush to collect data in an attempt to access these needs. I had great personal difficulty in finding out just what they were trying to measure. I suggested to one FHSA that they should ask general practitioners and district nurses on a regular basis what they thought patients needed, or even ask the patients themselves. However, as this would not produce an automatic system for informing the administration on how to distribute or re-allocate its resources, it was dismissed as Luddite.

Their approach to data collection was as follows:

> Firstly we collect the data, any data will do as long as it is data. We know it will not be accurate but we will use it in any case, and when the health care

professionals get their resources cut, they will soon react and tell us why the data is wrong and that will improve its accuracy.

This is of course a callous and now disreputable practice but because of this early attitude to data collection many health care professionals were demoralised, whilst others were infuriated, but they were all distracted from their main task of providing health care; a task in which they reasonably expected support from their administrative and managerial colleagues rather than the insensitivity and cynicism revealed by this approach. After a time, rather than expend the effort necessary to improve the accuracy of the data, health care professionals learn to provide data in a form that encourages the new administrative structure to give them more resources.

Finally a new equilibrium is reached as the administrative and managerial structures settle down, that assumes data accuracy is adequate now that everyone has learnt to play the new game.

The problems over data validity are fiercest in resource reallocation, because the information deduced from the data collected is used to take resources away from one area of activity and place them in another area where "gaps" have appeared. The abstracted deductions of management stimulate those who provide services to react unfavourably when their day to day experience does not tally with the central overview. The data on which management relies must be truly robust as it will inevitably be a source of conflict with those who have the task of actually reducing the volume or quality of the services they provide for patients.

Before the NHS was united, there was a tension between general practitioners outside the hospital wall, and the specialists within it. Those inside determined what they were going to provide for the problems that presented to them. They classified these problems into those that they could treat and solve or investigate, and those that were really part of another specialty which they could ignore. There was a third group of problems which were undefined or uninteresting, and belonged to the body of medicine known as general practice, and was out with the secondary care sector.

There were many unsatisfactory aspects of those tensions, but the disturbing new tension in the NHS is between the" Real" and "the Abstract". Previously tensions were between the reality of the hospital experience and the reality of general practice, and the interface was between one set of clinicians (and administrators) inside and another set of clinicians (and administrators) outside, each with different perspectives. Now with the unified NHS the tension is between the reality of all clinicians in practice and the theory of what government or purchasers wish to achieve. These theoretical targets have been clearly enunciated in the health of the nation targets as well as the more locally determined equivalents but the evidence for the theory has to be of at least equivalence to the evidence of practice. The evidence based medicine that is demanded of healthcare professionals must be matched by evidence based policies espoused by politicians and their functionaries.

8. Removal of "soft" advisory structures

The preceding section has stressed the importance of obtaining advice from those who collect data and who provide services. An unfortunate trend has been for management to obscure even further the difficulties and realities of practice by using selective rather than representative advice. The managerial excuse is that those who have been selected by the professions themselves to represent the views of the profession, will be more concerned with the vested interests of their profession rather than the patients they serve.

The progressive removal of doctors and other health care professionals from the administration over the last five or more years has accelerated. In the days of Executive Councils and FPC's virtually half of the authorities were drawn from the practising contractor professions. In the re-organisation of the NHS in 1974 reserved places for GP's, consultants and nurses on health authorities were retained, with well supported advisory structures for the various disciplines. The new internal market structures have virtually disbanded the "independent" networks within the structure, although following the Functions and Manpower Review[17] it was belatedly realised that there was still a need for professional advice by those who provide services.

Managers have frequently assumed the mantle of understanding and knowledge of healthcare professionals, but without having their training or competence. Management has often taken on the role of acting on behalf of patients, but without their consent or authority. Managers have not infrequently been given the task of prioritising and rationing cash limited services by politicians who have ducked this responsibility. It is no small wonder why those in NHS management find themselves unpopular and this unpopularity is compounded when they are selective in their search for professional advice.

A further difficulty faced by management structures is how to reconcile advice from different professional groups. The current fashion to only obtain multi-professional advice is an attempt to make sure that the health care professionals themselves resolve the inter-professional differences, rather than allow it to be a task of management. However there are times when pure medical advice is the driver for change despite the difficulties that it will bring in its wake for other health care professionals, and to channel all advice through multi-disciplinary advisory groups will bring its own inherent dangers.

9. Security of clinical information systems and network issues - Where do the problems lie?

It is quite clear that many of the current methods of recording and communicating carried out by GP's and hospital health care professionals do not meet the strict criteria of standards of security that is implicit in the GMC's Guidance on Confidentiality. For example, some GP's use a lap top computer to dial, via an open telephone line into their own practice database to look up and even alter the patient's records that are held at their surgeries. They may even contact the practice through an Internet node. It is more than likely that this is done without any access security checks or any encryption of the data flowing between the GP outside his surgery and the surgery records themselves. Practices such as these should cease, until the means of sending data securely from one location to another are in place.

However, it is not enough to ensure that the data is secure, but the identity of the person trying to access the database must be known and authorised by the practice. Whether some or all data is encrypted as it is entered into the computer or only as it leaves it or only after it is transmitted beyond the location where it is created needs to be determined.

Another question that surrounds present practice in hospitals is how many unknown and unidentified individuals have access to patient information. Leaving aside the obvious threats to confidentiality via illicit telephone enquiries, and just concentrating on the computerised records that are held, a large number of people have potential access to a large number of records within most hospital complexes. Currently many hospitals have open connection to external organisations, (for example computer suppliers who provide support to their computer systems) who can access confidential data simply because there are no security controls in place.

It has been proposed that both GP and hospital practices could be improved by an effective network[18]. For example the identity of anyone who dials into the network could be challenged, and the challenge would only allow an authorised GP to access his own database if he had been so identified. This is certainly better than the current practice of using telephone lines or the Internet.

It is proposed that the Codes of Connection that are described for the NWN (NHS Wide Network) will prevent hospitals with sloppy and insecure external connections from continuing to use them. They will not however do anything about the internal security, nor will they determine who can access each clinical record within that hospital. Any investment that only partially secures confidentiality must be judged inadequate and very poor value for money.

To ensure that individual patients data are protected, there must be external independent audit of all breaches of security, even to the extent that there should be unannounced challenges to systems to test if they are indeed secure. When any system is shown to be insecure, all patients whose records are held in that system should be notified.

Other IM&T projects such as NHS Administrative Registers and the National Clearing Service are considered essential for the internal market. Whether they continue or not will depend on how the NHS is managed and resourced in the future, and whether a less bureaucratic mechanism can be created. In the meantime these projects should not provide opportunities for undermining patients' rights to consent and confidentiality any further. Since patient consent and the confidentiality of personal health information are at the heart of the BMA's concerns, those who are responsible for the structure, functioning, and management of the infrastructure projects should be at pains to reassure healthcare professionals and the public on all accounts. Unsupported and unrepresentative professional membership of project boards is insufficient.

The BMA's security document addresses security in clinical information systems. The current poor levels of security of these systems are brought into sharp focus by the concept - rather than the reality - of the NWN. Whilst it must be frustrating to those who are trying their best to introduce security measures into a network which attempts to improve upon the security of the current networks that are used, they have failed to understand that the real problem that faces doctors and other health care professionals is the totality of security of the systems they use. A security policy that recognised this fact would not have adopted the NHS Executive's current strategy.

There is no question that the network issue has raised the profile of this debate. It has at last focused public attention upon the central questions of "informed consent", "need to know", and the actual security of the current systems that are being used in doctors' surgeries and hospitals.

The BMA's challenge now is to demonstrate how its security principles can be put into practical effect. Not only are there technical issues to be addressed, but careless administrative and professional habits and behaviour that have to radically change.

10. Trust and distrust, and fear of the future

Until approximately 18 months ago developments in computerised medical record systems were driven by enthusiasts in informatics. They were reassured by those who were driving the NHS strategy, particularly the security aspects of that strategy that all was well because there had always been an atmosphere of trust within practices and within hospitals, and in the majority of districts between clinicians and those in management. It was a difficult conceptual leap for many working in the NHS to accept that such trust could be misused. Indeed, the scenarios that have been drawn up in the recent public debate over the NWN could undermine doctors' belief in the trustworthiness of their professional and managerial colleagues, and in NHS employees as a whole. This sense of distrust may already have spilled over into the public's perception of how records in general are guarded within the NHS.

The only way that we can continue to practice medicine in any health care setting is by maintaining the trust that exists between patients and the health care professionals who are involved in their individual personal care. From henceforth this will only be possible if the systems that we use and the policies we adopt are indeed secure.

These concerns are not just confined to the United Kingdom. At a meeting of European general practitioners in Ireland on the 11 & 12 May 1996, UEMO (The European Union of General Medical Practitioners) endorsed the nine principles set out in the BMA policy document. To this was added a tenth, governing the question of data transfer.

> "The transfer of data must be secure and its integrity guaranteed. Encryption should occur to all data transmissions of clinical data when transmitted outside the location of the creation of that data".

The NHS Executive has responded to the BMA's wish to see clinical data encrypted by commissioning a report. Unfortunately, what is proposed as a trust structure for authorising the encryption keys (and by implication for controlling access to the data encrypted), does not reflect the traditional trust structures of clinical practice. The authorisation of access to a medical record should start with the subject of that record (ie, the patient) and the author of that record (usually the doctor or other healthcare professional).

Any transfer of the power for making such decisions of access to records away from the participants in consultation is unacceptable, even if it is done under the guise of a trusted third party for the purpose of improved security.

Many European doctors welcome the patient held smart card as a means for authorising access to the patient's own medical records. There are, however, opportunities for abusing even this safeguard by employers exerting unreasonable pressure on their employees to consent to their private medical record being revealed as a condition of employment. However, if access can only be gained with the simultaneous use of the doctor's key, such abuse can be minimised.

There is widespread European concern that those who seek to control healthcare expenditure, whether in government, insurance companies or sick funds are less concerned about the confidentiality and the consent of patients and more concerned about the efficiency and viability of their own organisations.

11. Conclusion

There are two temporal dimensions to a consideration of future issues.

One is for the present and predictable immediate future, when we should examine carefully what is proposed for guarding the security of our records and communications; And secondly, there is the more remote future when something that may be put in place now could be misused by those who will control the organisation in the future, perhaps less benevolent administrations or others with clear criminal intent.

Our priority must be to quantify the costs and time it will take to address the first set of issues. It is however important to keep a weather eye on more distant future dangers, which are at present unlikely possibilities, but the difficulties of building in counter measures for such eventualities should not be summarily dismissed.

With the passage of time the present remote future will become a more immediate reality and we will have to face new threats as they arise. We should therefore uphold the rights of every individual citizen to privacy.

Privacy is a continuum, through private thoughts to private behaviour. The consultation is a sanctum in which such intimate matters are declared and often recorded. Only when the privacy of this fundamental human activity is voluntarily breached by individual patients should it become a matter of public interest.

As a trusted guardian of such privacy, the doctor has an ethical duty to uphold the confidences revealed. A healthcare system that ignores or undermines this professional duty will be incapable of supporting the comprehensive care demanded by patients.

12. References

1. Lord Walton's Bill (Disclosure and Use of Personal Health Information). House of Lord's 2nd Reading - 13 March 1996.
2. "Security in Clinical Information Systems". (BMA). ISBN. 0727910485. 11 January 1996.
3. "Good Medical Practice". October 1995; Guidance from the General Medical Council.
4. Younger Committee on Privacy 1970-1972; Data Protection Committee: Sir NormanLindop.
5. Confidentiality of Personal Health Information. John Asbury. BMJ 1984. V289. P1559-60.
6. The Data Protection Act 1984: (1) A Code of Practice for General Medical Practitioners - March 1991; (2) Guidance to General Medical Practitioners on Data Protection Registration - June 1990. GMSC (BMA) Publication.
7. Statement to Committee Stage NHS Act 1990. Roger Freeman, Minister of Health. PHansard.
8. Quinquennial Cervical Smears: Every Woman's Right and Every General Practitioner's Responsibility. Standing P, Mercer S. BMJ. 6 October 1984, 289, 883-886.
9. Prevention of Cardiovascular Disease in General Practice: A Proposed Model. Angard EE, Land JM, Lenihan CJ, Packard CJ, Percy MJ, Ritchie LD, Shepherd J. BMJ Clinical Research 293(6540), 177-80, July 1986.
10. Proposed GP Fundholding Software Specifications: Comments - Jenkins SAP; GMSC Archives 1990.
11. The Philosophy of Investigation and Early Diagnosis: Jenkins SAP, September 1991. British Society of Gastroenterology - International Workshop on Early Gastric Cancer.
12. Keeping it in the Family. The Health Service Journal, 25 July 1991. Simon Jenkins No 5262, Vol 202, p35.
13. Safe Havens Offer Little Security. BMA News Review. June 1994. P31.
14. Steering Group on Health Services Information. Chairman: Mrs E Korner. Reports 1983-1985. Foundations for an Electronic Medical Record: AL Rector, WA Nowlan, S Kay. Meth. Inform. Med 1991, 30; 179-86.
15. Report of a Study of Family Practitioner Services Administration and the Use of Computers. Department of Health & Social Security. Welsh Office. Arthur Anderson. July 1984.
16. Steering Group on Health Services Information. Chairman: Mrs E Korner. Reports 1983-1985.
17. New High Command for the NHS. BMJ 1993. Vol 307. P1091.
18. (a) The Handbook of Information Security: Information Security within General Practice. Department of Health. May 1995. Ref E5209. NHSE. IMC. Birmingham B15 1JD
    (b) Information Systems Security: Top Level Policy for the NHS. Data Protection and Security. NHS. IMC. Birmingham B15 1JD.
    (c) Codes of Connection. IMG. E5222 & E5223.

Chances, Risks and Side Effects of Chip Cards in Medicine: A Technology Assessment Study from Germany

Anja Hartmann and Otto Ulrich*

Bundesamt fuer Sicherheit in der Informationstechnik (BSI)
Division for Technology Assessment
post box 200363, 53133 Bonn, Germany

1. Introduction

The social security organizations in Germany are confronted with a lot of problems. The costs are continously increasing, the receipts are steadily decreasing. The government has decided to reduce the benefits of the social security and to control the misuse of social services. That is why a bill against the "explosion of costs" has been prepared in the health ministry which became law in 1993.

Along with this law a "medical insurance card" has been introduced: each person is bound to submit the card in medical practices as well as in hospitals. This medical insurance card is a small card (similar to a credit or telephone cards) with a chip on it. The following data are stored on this chip card: the name of the insurance carrier, the name of the insured, his date of birth as well as his address, the insurance number of the policy holder, the beginning of the insurance coverage and at last the period of validity of the card. Two objectives are pursued with this card: the rationalization of administrative tasks in medical practices and in hospitals, and the proof of an insurance coverage of the patients (1, 2). To exclude any misuse of the medical insurance card, the manufacturers are bound to a technical specification concerning the card and the card reader. One of the requirements is that only the insurances shall be able to write, change or delete data on the cards. The "Bundesamt fuer Sicherheit in der Informationstechnik (BSI)" is evaluating the cards and card readers in regard to their information technology security (IT-security), and if passing the examination awards a certificate to the manufacturers. That is the status in 1996.

But the technical development of the medical insurance card is going on. Not only the manufacturers of chip cards and chip card readers, but also the health insurances, medical associations and scientists are thinking about further applicabilities (3). Depending on their different interests they plan to store various other types of data on the cards like treatment data (e.g. bills for medical treatment), emergency data (e.g. blood group, allergy, disease), blood donor and/or organ donor data, vaccination data, diagnostic data (e.g. cancer, diabetis), therapy data (e.g. operation, cure) or prescription data.

---

* This paper reflects the opinion of the authors only.

Such an extension of the medical insurance card towards a **patient card** is - depending on the design - combined with both progress and risks.

The supporters are pointing out that

- further costs could be saved,
- duplicate examinations could be avoided,
- in case of emergency, lifesaving data would be available as quickly as possible,
- the patients would not have to repeat their anamnesis to each physician they are visiting anew,
- the patients could hold their medical data themselves as the data is no longer stored in the different medical practices. (1)

On the other hand the antagonists are reminding again and again on the dangers:

- the communication flow between physicians and patients could deteriorate,
- the quantity of medical treatments as well as the quality of diagnosis and therapy could deteriorate,
- forwarding of data could occur without knowledge and consent of the patients,
- a lot of questions concerning data protection and data security are not yet known and even less solved. (4)

A lot of questions are arising which are not only concerning the "if, how and when" of the technological development, but also the consequences of various development potentials:

- Which risks are expected in case of appropriate use or in case of misuse of the patient cards?
- Who will decide how to judge opposite values, like security or economy in a conflicting situation?
- And last but not least: Who will take responsibility if somebody will be hurt? Who will be responsible for mistakes (manufacturers, physicians, others)?

2. Chip Cards in Medicine - the TA-Project of the German "Bundesamt fuer Sicherheit in der Informationstechnik (BSI)"

In February 1993 the German BSI has initiated a TA-project to analyze questions concerning IT-security in important applications of information technology like traffic, health systems, monetary system or process control. The project was being carried out by two German institutions: the "Industrieanlagen-Betriebsgesellschaft (IABG)" Ottobrunn and the "Fraunhofer Institute for System Technology and Innovation Research (FhG-ISI)" Karlsruhe, was completed in July 1994. The objectives of the discourse-project were

- to show the various stages of technological development,
- to analyze questions of security and vulnerability,
- to point out advantages as well as risks,
- to sensitize the different parties and
- to work out possible action.

The project was characterized by two very important approaches:

1. An interdisciplinary discourse was chosen to cope with the very complex task and to complement disciplinary knowledge. In addition, there was the requirement to bring together all persons concerned with the patient card, e.g. manufacturers, users, scientists and affected persons, ministry officials, data protectors, journalists and patients.
2. Scenarios were to be developed to illustrate the main problems of different design options (see below).

The first step was addressed to the problem of IT-security. Starting point of the discussion was the traditional concept of IT-security. This concept is based on the exclusion or reduction of dangers (5) and focusses on technical problems like operating errors, technical failures, failures caused by various types of disasters or manipulation attempts. But in the opinion of the discourse participants, the main technical demands like availability (prevention of the unauthorised withholding of information), integrity (prevention of the unauthorised modification of information) and confidentiality (prevention of the unauthorised disclosure of information) (5) were not far-reaching enough. Therefore it has been agreed that a more comprehensive concept of IT-security including social, legal and economical elements should be taken as a basis.

A technology assessment concerning questions of IT-security therefore has to include the following examination levels:

- technical and technological elements of IT-security, i.e. availability, integrity and confidentiality,
- organizational elements, e.g. questions concerning the medical documentation,
- legal and economical elements, i.e. questions of legal compatibility and efficiency, as well as
- social and ecological elements, i.e. questions of social vulnerability and dependence on workable information technology.

In this context the legal compatibility is one of the main demands on the design of secure IT-systems.

2.1 Scenarios Concerning the Design of Chip Cards in Medicine

To assess the consequences of the use of chip cards in medicine the following questions were of elementary interest:

- which are the main technologies for the technical design of a patient card? We have to distinguish between (6,7,8):
  - storage chip cards
  - processor cards
  - smart cards
  - optical cards
  - .....

- which types of data in the health system are relevant for an electronical use? On the agenda are:
  - data of the membership fee
  - treatment data
  - blood donor or organ donor data
  - vaccination data
  - diagnostic data
  - therapy data or
  - prescription data.

The main reasons for the introduction of a patient chip card are the improvement of the medical care, i.e. the 'quality of care', and the increased visibility of treatments. The participants of the discourse decided to focus the project on the following types of data: treatment data, diagnostic data and therapy data.

- which actors are involved in the development, storing, forwarding or changing of data? The health system in Germany shows a wide range of actors, who could be interested in the data stored on the chips:
  - patients
  - physicians
  - working doctors
  - hospitals
  - medical associations
  - health insurances
  - drugstores
  - medical services
  - scientists
  - ......

The interweaving of the mentioned components results in a complex matrix of design options, which have been checked to see whether they are lawful or not. The resulting, very reduced matrix has then to be linked with the starting question: which problems concerning IT-security are combined with which individual configuration? And: what can be done or which precautions are helpful to raise the security level?

Falling back on the technical elements of IT-security we can distinguish between various security levels:

- a low security level is regarded as sufficient if the protection can be limited (restricted) to operating errors and/or the arising possible damage is rated low (e.g. medical insurance card, chip card with treatment data),
- a medium security level is required if there is an increased potential for damages (e.g. chip card with therapy data) and/or it must be reckoned on manipulation attempts,
- a high security level is necessary, if we have to count on wide-range or long-term damages in case of technical failures, manipulation attempts, operating errors or failures caused by various disasters. The demand for this security level is stronger as more medical data are to be stored on the patient card. Malfunction or loss of data can result in wrong decisions of the physicians and in disastrous consequences for the patients (ultimately to the death). (9)

When the participants of the discourse constructed the scenarios, they attached great importance to build one scenario for each of the mentioned security levels. Background for this was the hypothesis, that depending on the various dangers, there could be a need for different action to increase the security of a patient card. The following scenarios have been discussed:

- "patient chip card with treatment data", which will be used for the account of treatments with health insurances;
- "patient chip card with diagnostic data", which will serve for the medical check-up and treatment. This card is considered as particulary dangerous, because both unauthorized access (e.g. of the employer) and the loss of data (e.g. the information that a pregnant woman has AIDS) can result in far-reaching consequences for patients as well as for physicians and medical assistants;
- "patient chip card with therapy data", which will also serve for the medical treatment, but where the potential damage is estimated lower.

2.2 Resulting Possible Action

The options can be associated to the above mentioned examination levels of IT-security. In the following presentation we have to take into consideration, that the results of the interdisciplinary discourse-project are preliminary - further refinement is necessary. There is a common consensus concerning the various action potentialities, but opinions differ in regard to their classification according to the above mentioned types of cards and data. Some participants of the discourse call for the implementation of the whole range of options, while others propose a ranking of various options according to the different damage potentials.

Discussed options concerning the technical examination level

In Europe as well as in the United States and Japan there is a scientific and political discussion about the application of different levels of IT-security. Seven Levels from E0 (low) to E7 (very high) are distinguished. The options concerning the technical examination are therefore oriented by the criteria for IT-security "ITSEC" (10):

- scenario 1: a patient chip card with treatment data should reach the level E2/E3,
- scenario 2: a patient chip card with diagnostic data needs a very high security level, so E4/E5 is necessary,
- scenario 3: the damage potential of a patient chip card with therapy data is in between those of scenario 1 and 2. Therefore an IT-security level of E3/E4 suffices.

Discussed options concerning the organizational examination level

In the context of the organizational examination level we have discussed those options which are resulting from medicine or medical informatics and have direct consequences for the patients:

- questions concerning the medical documentation. At the moment every physician is taking his notes according to his personal preferences. There is up to now no standardized scheme for medical documentation in Germany. The physicians neither have guidelines nor the International Code of Diseases (ICD) may be used. The introduction of the International Code of Diseases (ICD) in Germany have been put on the back burner until 1998. Some german interest groups remind the politicians and the health insurances of the dangers. Especially the Codes for homosexuality and for mental diseases are controversial. So the ICD have to be revised. The discussion on the ICD illustrates the problematic nature of standardization of medical documentation. Scenario 2 or 3 can not be implemented without any standarization. and medical data can hardly be stored on chips.

- questions concerning data protection. The patient must be able to recognize, who has which rights to access, and when and why physicians or other persons are changing, processing, forwarding or deleting data.
- questions concerning the relations between chip cards and existing networks. For example: If there is not enough capacity on a chip card to store large data (e.g. computer tomography), the patients should be able to chose, whether the physician may access the stored data via network or not.

Discussed options concerning the legal examination level

The participants of the discourse demand the examination of each scenario concerning both, the legal compatibility (at the moment the lawyers in Germany do not consider the scenarios 2 and 3 as lawful) and an implementation of the design criteria developed by BIZER (11):

- The patients should be able to decide on their own, whether they want to use a chip card, which kind of data will be stored on the card and when the data will be deleted.
- The stored data may only be used for a defined purpose, e.g. medical treatment, medical account or - in an anonymous form - for scientific work.
- Only those data may be stored, which are absolutely necessary for physicians and medical assistants. As already mentioned above, there is no standard for medical documentation in Germany. In case the medical chip card is introduced there is a great need for rules concerning the medical documentation.
- The patients are entitled to inspect the stored data, whenever they want. Patients must always be able to read the stored data as well as to fathom changing and processing of data. From the patients' point of view visiblity is one of the most important demands.
- There must be security precautions against unauthorized access; e.g,. employers, insurances, heirs and scientists should not be able to access the data in any way.
- There must be some rules about the responsibility in case of failures. Who is responsible in case of a malfunction of the chip card or chip card reader, or in case of an unauthorized access? The authenticity and intactness of the data has to be guarantied.

Discussed options concerning the social examination level

The social discussion concerning the use of chip cards in the health system is up to now highly influenced by economical arguments. The physicians should be able to gain time in the inquiry of the anamnesis. In addition, costs could be reduced, because duplicate examinations can be avoided. In this context the patients are afraid that the communication flow between physicians and patients could deteriorate and that they don't know enough about the patient card, the various possibilities to use the card and the dangers.

The following options result from the considerations:

- The introduction and use of a patient chip card have to be accompanied by comprehensive informations. We have to qualify patients and other affected persons about their rights and the possibilities and risks of the card.
- We have to take measures against the deterioration of the relations between patients and physicians, e.g. the doctors have to be trained in forms of conversation.
- The patients should be able to visit a second physician without telling him the diagnosis of his colleague.
- All concerned persons together have to develop an advanced security culture (12). What does it mean? Each person has an individual need for security. The more sensitive the data are the greater is this need. Out of this need of security various social groups develop different collective manners to handle insecurity, threats and risks.

  In the example "Chip Cards in Medicine" the need for security is extraordinary high for patients (because the risks for their health are very high), high for doctors (because they could lose patients if they did not consider the needs) and relatively low for a doctors' association (because their risks are reduced to legal questions).

  The different collective manners of all social groups affected by a technique result in the so called security culture. In addition, the security culture is caused by social learning processes. It is expressed by a specific perception and coping with reality. So, security measures, instructions and norms as well as informal methods are signs of a security culture. The security culture with regard to a specific technique is embedded in a social, economic and legal surrounding. Therefore it is influenced by several experiences persons have.

  The management of IT-security will only be successful, if the development of a security culture is adequately supported. It would indicate that communication and cooperation potentials concerning IT-security are practiced. As a result we found the phenomenon that IT-security is dependent on the organization of an interculturel communication and cooperation process (13). The advantage from this point of view is that we have the chance to use security culture as a junction between the great demand of IT-security and its reality (14).

So far the discussed options. Within the limitation of a small and short discourse project two problems had been tackled: all affected persons discussed together the pros and cons of various design options and a lot of unsolved questions arised (and for some of them there are suggested solutions). It had be seen that it was not possible to find answers to all of the arising questions. There are up to now still a lot of different opinions concerning the design options of a patient card. And there are also concerned persons that do not like a chip card at all.

The project was completed in July 1994. What happens afterwards? It is not in the responsibility of the Bundesamt fuer Sicherheit in der Informationstechnik (BSI) to make a political decision. The only thing the BSI can do is to inform the decisive persons. Therefore the results of the study had not only been published, but also discussed with some policy makers (e.g. in the german health ministry), manufacturers, interest groups, scientists and so on. It wasn't without some consequences: some of the scientists as well as some manufacturers includes various suggestions in their further work. The health ministry decided that the development and introduction of patient chip cards with diagnosis and therapy data on it is not derserve to be promoted in a special way. Nevertheless the german industry as well as some health insurances and interest groups try very hard to introduce the patient chip card. We notice various field tests and can only hope that they reflect the results of the above represented study.

Literature

(1) Schaefer, O.P., 1993: Die Versichertenkarte - Auftakt zu neuen Kommunikationsstrukturen im Gesundheitswesen. In: Datenschutz und Datensicherung, No. 12, pp.685-688.

(2) Kilian, Wolfgang, 1992: Legal Issues in Relation to Medical Chipcards. In: Köhler, C.O. (ed.): Cards, Databases and Medical Communication. Fourth Global Congress on Patient Cards and Computerization of Health Records, Berlin, Newton, Mass.: Medical Records Institute, 1992, pp. 53-53xii..

(3) Waegemann, C. Peter, 1992: The State-of-the-Art of Patient Cards - A Global View of Developments in the Field of Patient Cards and Computerisation of Health Records. In. Köhler, C.O. (ed.): Cards, Databases and Medical Communication. Fourth Global Congress on Patient Cards and Computerization of Health Records, Berlin, Newton, Mass.: Medical Records Institute, 1992, pp. 78-78ix.

(4) Kuhlmann, Jan, 1993: Die Verarbeitung von Patientendaten nach dem SGB V und das Recht auf selbstbestimmte medizinische Behandlung. In: Datenschutz und Datensicherung, No. 4, pp. 198-208.

(5) Kersten, Heinrich, 1992a: Neue Aufgabenstellungen des Bundesamtes fuer Sicherheit in der Informationstechnik. In: Datenschutz und Datensicherung, No. 6, pp. 293-297.

(6) Bundesamt fuer Sicherheit in der Informationstechnik (BSI), 1995: Chipkarten im Gesundheitswesen. Schriftenreihe des BSI, Band 5. Bonn.

(7) Köhler, Claus O,. 1993: Medizinische Dokumentation auf der Chipkarte - Eine neue Dimension. In: Quintessenz, No. 6, pp.627-633.

(8) Waegemann, Peter, 1993: Patient Card Technologies and Applications. In: Waegemann, Peter (ed.): Toward an Electronic Patient Record '93 - Ninth Annual International Symposium on the Computerization of Medical Records and North American Conference on Patient Cards, Newton, Mass., USA: Medical Record Institute, 1993, pp.175-178.

(9) Wellbrock, Rita, 1994: Chancen und Risiken des Einsatzes maschinenlesbarer Patientenkarten. In: Datenschutz und Datensicherung, No. 2, pp.70-74.

(10) Kersten, Heinrich, 1992b: Die Kriterienwerke zur IT-Sicherheit - ihre Bedeutung fuer die Anwendungspraxis. In: Wirtschaftsinformatik, No. 4, pp.378-390.

(11) Bizer, Johann, 1994: Rechtliche Möglichkeiten und Schranken der Patientenchipkarte. In: BSI 1994: Chipkarten in der Medizin. Dokumentation eines Fachdiskurses am 2. und 3. Dezember 1993 in Bad Aibling. BSI 7154. Bonn, pp.57-78.

(12) Hartmann, Anja, 1995: Sicherheitskultur zur Prävention vor Risiken und Nebenwirkungen des Chipkarteneinsatzes. In: Bundesamt für Sicherheit in der Informationstechnik (ed.): Patienten und ihre computergerechten Gesundheitsdaten. Interdisziplinärer Diskurs zu querschnittlichen Fragen der IT-Sicherheit. Ingelheim, pp 21-31.

(13) Ulrich, Otto, 1995: Sicherheitskultur im Gesundheitswesen einer modernen Demokratie. In: Blobel, Bernd (ed.): Datenschutz in medizinischen Informationssystemen. Braunschweig, pp.75-84.

(14) Hartmann, Anja, 1995: "Comprehensive Information Technology Security": A New Approach to Respond Ethical and Social Issues Surrounding Information Security in the 21st Century. In: Eloff, Jan/Solms von, Sebastian (ed.): Information Security - the next Decade. London 1995, pp. 590 - 602.

Exceptionalism Redux: How Different Is Health Care Informatics?

Reid Cushman

Yale University,
New Haven, Connecticut, USA
reid.cushman@yale.edu

> [T]he tremendous growth of computerized health data, the development of huge data banks and the advancements in record linkage, pose an enormous threat to the privacy of medical information. The public is generally unaware of this threat or of the serious consequences of a loss of confidentiality in the health care system. Adequate measures to control medical privacy, in light of the electronic information processing, can and must be established....
> (American Medical Record Association, 1974)

> [M]edical records shall be confidential, secure, current, authenticated, legible and complete. (Joint Commission on the Accreditation of Hospitals, 1976)

1. Health care exceptionalism

[1] Health care is different. Its exceptional characteristics, and the implications of that character for both equity and efficiency, are a perennial theme in a variety of literatures. Political economists since at least Adam Smith have stressed the special nature of "human capital investments" like health and education, which set the foundation for life's activities (Blaug, 1978). Consistent with this view, most industrialized nations have adopted policies that aim to reduce disparities in health services distribution. Some elevate health care access to the status of a constitutional principle, and employ the language of human rights. Even in the US, a last bastion of predominantly private health care finance, recent surveys show the populace continues to hold exceptionally egalitarian notions about health care (Schlesinger and Lee, 1993).

[2] Modern political economists, such as Kenneth Arrow (1963), have looked at the exceptional prevalence of uncertainty and "information imperfections" in health markets. (See Pauly, 1978, for a somewhat contrary view.) Consumers' uncertainty about their need for health care in future periods implies a strong role for insurance, be it socially-funded or private. Insurance mechanisms' inherent separation of consumption from price alter consumers' behavior in potentially inefficient ways (e.g., the "moral hazard" problem of excessive use). Consumers generally do not know the expected outcome of various treatments, and must rely on producers' advice — an "agency" relationship. Sometimes the producers themselves can only roughly predict outcomes, risks and benefits for an increasingly complex "product"; in general, though, the agents have the upper hand. The incentives inherent in particular reimbursement arrangements, coupled

with such information problems, give producers license to behave in inefficient ways as well (e.g., the "supplier-induced demand" problem).

[3] The US has had a particularly hard time translating its notions of health care equity into system-wide reform. On the efficiency side of the problem, however, there is frenetic activity aimed at promoting "correct" behavior: structures of copayments and deductibles for consumers; a balancing amongst fee-for-service, capitation, salary and incentive regimes for producers; all manner of market "intermediary" institutions. World-wide, there is a fervid quest for better information about the costs and benefits associated with the available range of drugs, devices and procedures, so that the "correct" rates of application can be known. Limited attention to such technology assessment — particularly of the "is this worth what it costs" variety — was until rather recently another element of health care's exceptionalism. High rates of expenditure growth helped end insouciance about value. So did the embarrassing discoveries of large variations in practice, such as by Wennberg in the US, which forced the industry to confront that there was "insufficient evidence" about the "diagnostic, therapeutic, and ultimate health effects" of many of its interventions (Institute of Medicine, 1990). Now an "outcomes research" sub-industry has sprung up to evaluate better both effectiveness and effectiveness relative to expense. And the regime known as "managed care" is built on an efficiency religion.

[4] Like most faiths, managed care and outcomes research have their extremist practitioners (and their unpleasant rituals), but they still arguably present a net improvement over the old "medicine is too much an art to be judged by economics" exceptionalist school. A society that considers health services exceptionally important — and understands the many impediments to efficiency — is duty-bound to pursue knowledge about whether its health services resources are wisely spent.

2. Information technology exceptionalism

[5] New information technology (IT) applications are expected to play a key role in reducing the knowledge deficit. As readers here are well aware, large-scale aggregations of computer-based clinical and administrative records are presumed to be a growing source of data for outcomes research. Database and decision-support tools, interfacing with electronic patient records, may someday be a principal mechanism by which research results are fed back into clinical choices. (See Institute of Medicine, 1991 and 1994, for more detail.) It is thus ironic that health care IT itself sometimes seems to be a last bastion of the old-style technology assessment exceptionalism which it will be used to eradicate. Great claims are not uncommonly made for new "automated" systems, without much clear proof of the magnitude of benefits, and with sometimes limited attention to the explicit and implicit costs. For example, the Institute of Medicine's otherwise comprehensive report, *The Computer-Based Patient Record: An Essential Technology for Health Care*, gives short shrift to matters of cost: "likely to be substantial but ... difficult to estimate," it concludes (Institute of Medicine, 1991). In most settings outside health care, the "essentialness" of a good depends considerably on the price tag.

[6] Recent estimates indicate the explicit price will indeed be substantial — tens of billions of dollars a year in the US alone, just for the computer and telecommunications

infrastructure. Yet the more important cost may be the implicit one, if these systems cannot be made secure. Given the volatile personal information commonly embedded in health records, an atmosphere of distrust about the security of computer-resident data inevitably breeds fears of personal humiliation, loss of reputation, and risks to financial status. This is particularly so in the US, where weak anti-discrimination and privacy protections coincide with the strong discriminatory incentives of private finance. In treatment settings, such fears may cause persons to increasingly withhold sensitive information from their health care providers. Such non-disclosure presents obvious risks for the patient, since it could materially affect the course of care. Equally, physicians may feel forced into keeping some types of data out of patient records (or into keeping duplicate, private records of sensitive information). Incomplete or inaccurate records have the potential to contaminate the knowledge base for outcomes research and surveillance. Sorting out privacy and security requirements is thus not just an engineering puzzle or an ethical "nicety," but a matter that potentially conditions the abilities of the clinical and research apparati of health care to perform appropriately.

[7] What do we know of the efficiency, broadly-defined, of the IT systems themselves? Even techno-enthusiasts admit that performance predictions for unprecedentedly large, ambitious information system designs are sometimes wide of the mark. Consider the US military's difficulties in implementing its own $2.8 billion world-wide EMR/CPR system (General Accounting Office, 1996). Or ponder the dark comedy of efforts to replace IT underlying the US air traffic control system (Wald, 1996). IT benefits specifications can be elusive even when the design mark is hit. Productivity and investment return are notoriously difficult to measure for computer and telecommunications investments, particularly in service industries like health care. "Payoffs ... are likely to be uncertain in both scale and timing ... [e]xpected value is often not quantifiable or even estimable, let alone predictable" (National Research Council, 1994). These frustrating incertitudes have often led to limited or nonexistent IT cost-benefit analyses. US government IT cost-benefit practice has been notably lackluster, despite the requirements of law and regulation (Regan, 1995).

[8] In the case of EMR/CPR systems, improved clinical decision-making logically flows from faster access to richer patient-specific data. Yet the fraction of patients for whom the improvement will be substantial, particularly enough to justify the large associated costs, is not yet known. Very sick, intensively-cared-for patients in hospital environments represent a paradigmatic case. So does the "emergency" patient, acutely ill and far from home, and with a complex medical history. Could we serve such cases equally well with intra-institutional EMRs, distributed data vehicles like smart cards, and a regime of only very limited networking? On the research side, the ultimate usability and cost of outcomes research data, derived from large-scale records mining, is also unclear (Institute of Medicine, 1990). Public-health-oriented "surveillance" may well be assisted substantially (Gostin et al, 1996). But hopes that such data amalgamations will be a cheap, high-quality substitute for controlled trials have to date not been realized (Office of Technology Assessment, 1994). Could we perhaps make do with less exhaustive, more focused databases? Could we preserve a strong right for patients to "opt out," without unacceptable compromise to data quality?

[9] Given the potentially large risks and the as-yet speculative scale of benefits, one might expect a cautionary, experimental approach to such questions. Instead, cradle-to-

grave records, with nationally- and even globally-networked health databanks constitute the modal plan. The prevailing belief is that the medical benefits of such systems outweigh security risks, and that the health sector is too far behind in its "automation" to go slow now. That belief may be correct, but it seems grounded on rather thin empirical evidence. Moreover, we know little about the actual state of health care information systems security today, about the nature and scope of both legal and illegal information traffic, or about the discriminatory behaviors that occur based on that information. In short, we have a limited "threat model" on which to ground systems design, even though we have seen the problem coming for a long time (see, e.g., Hiller and Beyda, 1981). One version of the "exceptionalism" question is precisely on whom the burden of proof should now fall, given the risks. Must IT systems first achieve some level of "safety and effectiveness" in the manner of a new drug? Or can we proceed apace until a lack of safety is proved? The default now seems to be the latter.

[10] For health care generally, technology assessment lagged behind sector growth in part because of historical factors: Until late in this century, practitioners could offer few interventions, fewer still that did much good; nothing cost very much, at least as measured by today's standards; and reimbursement regimes provided little incentive for self-discipline. Yet practitioners now pay a steep price for their technology assessment failings. Controls have been increasingly imposed from the "outside," by public and private payors, in sometimes very unpleasant ways. Health care IT applications have lagged behind sector growth as well, especially compared to industries like banking and finance, with isolated systems and limited functionality the norm. Now that the sector is "catching up" it should resist the temptation to give short shrift to careful assessment of IT itself. Information technology's importance as a "leveraging" technology for other efficiencies, its significant monetary costs, and its implications for privacy and discrimination, all argue for flinty-eyed technology assessment.

3. Practitioners' views: one example

[11] Instead, a certain Panglossian tendency characterizes many IT evaluations. Consider an article in the March/April 1996 edition of the *Journal of the American Medical Informatics Association,* entitled "Privacy, Confidentiality and Electronic Medical Records," by Randolph Barrows, Jr., MD and Paul Clayton, PhD. The authors are affiliated with the Center for Medical Informatics at Columbia-Presbyterian Medical Center (New York), an institution renowned for its advanced implementations of health care information systems. JAMIA itself is aimed, by its own description, at a readership oriented to "the practice of informatics." Given such a pedigree, the article must be taken seriously as evidence of the ethos and aspirations of persons who actually implement and administer electronic health data regimes, at least in the US. The attention of such an audience for privacy and confidentiality concerns is surely welcome.

[12] Barrows and Clayton laudably emphasize the importance of trust and confidentiality in health care interactions, and the critical need for preservation of both. They discuss the "significant economic, psychologic, and social harm that can come" when personal information is disclosed, and briefly itemize the "incomplete and inconsistent" current legal protections for privacy in the US. While "applicable security

technologies exist," borrowed from the banking and military sectors, the authors note that "experience is lacking" about the transferability and effectiveness of these regimes for the health environment. They discuss the intolerance within many health care facilities of inconveniences associated with security practices, and remark that even their own institution had difficulty making sound administrative policies to complement technical safeguards. Indeed, though Columbia-Presbyterian appears to be a model of good IT security, the authors note that many institutions could not meet the proposed 1995 information management standards of the Joint Commission on Accreditation of Health Care Organizations. Consequently, the JCAHO requirements were "downsized" with the "stated intention of a more gradual deployment."

[13] While "awareness of risks and of possible technical solutions is increasing," the authors would appear to be describing a rather precarious environment, at least in the short run. The picture does not improve when one focuses on the details of some of the technical fixes. Barrows and Clayton deem "tight" prospective access restrictions — a "need to know," mandatory access control model — as largely incompatible with the dynamic health care environment. Columbia-Presbyterian itself implements a limited access control matrix (classifying users as attending physicians, residents, medical students, hospital nurses, and so forth), with differing access privileges granted for each group. But the authors admit this offers fairly limited protection given the large number of users in each category: "[P]rohibition of access by most medical users to most data on most patients is often not practical," they say. Instead the security model is based on "need-to-show" controls, with users disciplined by the potential requirement to demonstrate, after the fact, why their access to a particular patient's information was appropriate.

[14] Good post-hoc need-to-show security requires an appropriate audit-trail facility, whereby significant system events are logged. Since such logging data are voluminous, they must be analyzed by computer-based techniques to have a reasonable chance of detecting problems; no human could parse them unassisted. And what of such tools?

> Statistical techniques lend themselves to anomaly detection but are inadequate to detect all types of intrusions and do not prevent users from gradually training their usage profiles, so that activity previously considered anomalous might be regarded as normal. Expert-systems and model-based techniques lend themselves to misuse detection, but specification of the ordering on facts, for the pattern matching of events, has been deleteriously inefficient.... Each system is out of necessity ... somewhat ad hoc and custom designed.... *[N]o commercially available audit-analysis tool kit yet exists, and there is as yet no known application of software tools for audit analysis in the health care sector.* (Barrows and Clayton, 1996; emphasis added)

After the basic mechanics of identification and authentication (e.g., by user-ids and passwords), event-logging and audit are the most important line of defense against access violations. But at least for now, in health care, it would seem to be a weak line.

[15] The situation is little better with encryption. Barrows and Clayton note that "for practical purposes, due to the embedding of sensitive data in text objects" all health data should be encrypted. Encryption is also essential for assuring that data is uncorrupted and that it came from the expected source (message accuracy and authentication,

respectively). Again, however, there is a critical problem of technology availability. Cheap, effective cryptographic hardware and software have been slow to appear on the market, in part because of uncertainties about government export controls (Office of Technology Assessment, 1995).

> Software tool kits for the secure transmission and archiving of files by medical applications are beginning to appear. In the near future, vendor products will supply encryption technology embedded within computer systems for health care. Until then, [EMR] developers are forced to create their own implementations of well-known and secure cryptographic algorithms and protocols.... *Cryptographic techniques applicable to the goals of privacy, integrity and access control have not yet been significantly deployed in the health care environment, and experience is needed before establishing that they could provide security solutions compatible with the diversity of health care needs.* (Barrows and Clayton, 1996; emphasis added)

As with audit trail mechanisms, a requirement for ad hoc implementation usually guarantees a low rate of utilization, since one-off designs are expensive (and requisite expertise can be unavailable at any price). Thus it is perhaps unsurprising that Ernst & Young's 1995 information security survey found only about one-quarter of some 1300 reporting US institutions regularly used encryption to protect data. The rate for the 134 health care respondents in the survey was even less impressive: only one in ten.

[16] Given a precarious legal environment, a lagging and arguably recalcitrant institutional environment, and on-going availability and implementation deficits for critical security technologies, one might conclude there is cause for concern and a lot of caution. Barrows and Clayton conclude: "[S]ubstantial advantages to the electronic record exist, and it seems prudent to move ahead with implementations of electronic records." We may worry that the real conjunction in this sentence is a "therefore," not an "and" — the vision of "substantial advantages" pressing the notion of "prudence." In my dictionary, the latter defined as:

> 1. The state, quality or fact of being prudent. 2. Careful management; economy.... Synonyms: *prudence, discretion, circumspection.* These nouns are compared as they express caution and wisdom in the conduct of affairs. *Prudence*, the most comprehensive, implies not only caution but the capacity for judging in advance the probable results of one's actions.... (emphasis in original)

This is precisely what devotees of EMR systems cannot currently offer, given the many uncertainties.

4. Relative risks: paper vs electrons

[17] To be sure, security with paper systems has rarely been remarkably good, despite the long-standing requirements of certification bodies like JCAHO. Indeed, this is something proponents of EMRs almost always bring up in short order. Paper's typical problems are well known: inadequate access validation and "logging" procedures by file clerks, to control and trace which records are sent where; defective physical security for central repositories, and for individual records as they move within and among

institutions; the omnipresence of the photocopier and fax machine to reproduce documents (Office of Technology Assessment, 1993). While this may be a partial defense of moving on to electronic systems, which at least will (someday) afford facilities like audit-trails to trace use, it also raises an interesting counter-question. Why have so few moved authoritatively to rectify the "glaring" security problems with paper records? The answer seems to be that such protection has not been considered worthy of serious attention — or, more accurately, serious money. Information access has been the priority.

[18] Attitudes change a lot more slowly than does technology. We may presume that access considerations will still trump security concerns, in many institutions, as the sector moves to predominantly electronic environments. At least they seem likely to do so absent new legal or regulatory pressures. Barrows and Clayton remark that "[e]lectronic medical records are arguably more secure [than paper] if the proper policies and best available technologies are in place." Perhaps they mean the best soon-to-be-available technologies, but even granting the premise does not end the matter. First, unlike the place the authors inhabit, most institutions will likely be far behind the "best practices." In a networked world, security is often only as good as the weakest institutional link. While high-quality empirical data is lacking, there is ample reason to suspect that the average level of IT security in health care institutions is not very good and, given deficits in expertise and monetary resources, the situation is likely to improve only slowly. (See Ernst & Young, 1995a and 1995b; Riley, 1996; and discussion below.)

[19] Second, even an accurate "average" figure by itself tells only part of the story, given the clearly different risk structures. Paper records carry high probabilities of small (individual record) violations, but low probabilities of large breaches given the physical difficulties of manipulation. Electronic environments inevitably carry significant non-zero probabilities of large information losses, once a security breach has occurred. The risk structure is roughly analogous to that for production of electric power. Fossil-fuel plants, by virtue of the pollutants they produce, impose a small but almost certain adverse health effect on populations surrounding the generating plant. Nuclear power plants may obviate this low-end risk, but bring a non-zero probability of catastrophic consequences of the Chernobyl kind. (The problem of long-term waste disposal raises yet another important risk difference.) Whatever one's view on the comparative merits of these alternative approaches to alternating current, very rarely does one focus on the mean risk when contemplating a choice between them.

[20] Information leaks are not quite of the same class as radiation leaks, of course, though they share the characteristic of being very difficult to clean up after they've occurred. And for either, one dramatic leak, whatever its actual consequences, has the possibility of substantially eroding the public's confidence. Trust is not an asset in particularly robust supply in today's rapidly changing health systems. It will be a great irony indeed if information technology, intended to "save" health care by pointing a way toward greater efficiency, ends up substantially undermining the trust essential to system functioning.

5. Ludditism vs prudence

[21] Only a true Luddite would advocate standing pat with paper until "absolute" security can be achieved. There is, of course, no such animal. The rational question is one of marginal adjustments — here, whether we should reduce the rate, scale or scope of IT implementations given safety concerns. Security is expensive, and has no natural constituency. When resources are tight, we know it is commonly a casualty. Even in the best of times, careers may not be advanced by the hypothetical counterfactual "if we hadn't had good systems security, then we would probably have experienced more/some system breaches." Hospitals are the logical epicenter of EMR/CPR implementations, with inter-hospital and inter-system networking following. In the US, hospitals are under tremendous competitive pressure as the industry restructures under managed care (e.g., to a much greater level of out-patient services). Mergers, consolidations and closures are expected to continue. Reimbursement levels from both private payers and government are continually ratcheting downward, narrowing profit margins for the surviving institutions. It would be hard to describe an environment less likely to have the discretionary resources for an investment in robust data security — even for current systems, much less ambitious new ones.

[22] Beyond anecdotes, though, what hard evidence do we have about current threats? Not much. But the limited data provides little comfort. Consider that in the 1995 Ernst & Young survey, 57 percent of the health care institutions responding reported an information security-related loss in the last two years, up from 54 percent in the preceding year's survey. (For all respondents, the figures were 54 percent and 53 percent, respectively.) Some 88 percent of the health care institutions considered that their security risks were worsening (85 percent for all respondents). Even granting that such responses may lump together both the negligible and the serious, those are high numbers. (Out of circumspection or simple inability, most respondents declined to estimate the dollar value of their losses.) The survey's data on security practices is just as unsettling. Health care respondents had on average very low rates of technical security measures (such as encryption). Health facilities also had low rates of complementary administrative practice (e.g., security awareness and training programs). Despite this, health care institutions had a higher level of satisfaction with their own security effectiveness than any other industry included in the survey. With all the health sector's recent difficulties, it's at least good to know that self-esteem isn't a problem too.

6. Real informed consent?

[23] In a western health care environment whose foremost paradigm is patient autonomy, the slogan of "informed consent" is regularly brought forth. Applied to the IT environment, it can be thought of as requiring that patients be given the clear opportunity to "opt out" of certain kinds of uses and disclosures of their data, or more generally to decline permission for their health information to be stored in the full range of electronic repositories. While clinicians and researchers rarely snub their noses at autonomy per se, it is rare to find one who is cheery about letting patients routinely escape from the usual and customary databanks. It's too inconvenient. Too costly. Too disruptive. Potentially compromising to research. Et cetera. Indeed, it is probably all of these things. We

should be glad that it is, for only inconvenience, cost, and the odd lawsuit are likely to focus the mind on patients' preferences for credible security. In a world where patients are routinely forced to sign blanket waivers, allowing virtually any sort of subsequent storage and distribution, there is no such discipline.

[24] Even with the most nuanced of waiver forms, though, informed consent must be more fiction than fact for the average patient. In a system like the US's, opting out is at best an option only for those who can afford to self-pay. Given the expense associated with most medical treatments, that is a small fraction. Moreover, almost any encounter generates information, no matter who pays. You can't get care at all unless you are willing to divulge symptoms (which enter a history file); treatments inevitably generate data sequelae too (e.g., in order-entry or pharmacy systems). Really opting out requires not just wealth but the willingness to seek care under a pseudonym — hardly a realistic option for most. Codes of ethics such as the AMA's (1994) can require that practitioners apprise patients of the uses to which their data will be put (for the "informed" part of consent). But most providers probably don't know enough about information practices to tell patients anything coherent — beyond a sort of vague medical version of the US criminal law's Miranda warning — in the rare instances that the question is posed.

[25] Information practices are, like almost everything else that transpires within a health system encounter, as much a matter of "uninformed trust" as informed consent. (Cynics may say "semi-informed distrust" is a more accurate characterization.) Persons walk freely into care settings — if well enough to walk — but generally they no more pass judgment on the safety and appropriateness of the arrangements than does the average person stepping onto an elevator or a jet airplane.

[26] In the clinical setting, patients in theory give informed consent to any and all treatments offered by practitioners. If they are incapable of competent assent, authorized proxy decision-makers (a relative or a friend) do so in their stead. But we know that the medical environment is inevitably one of substantial "information asymmetry." Patients rarely have the expertise to assess the diagnoses and treatment options offered by the practitioner. They must place trust in the technical skills and personal motivations of their "agent." It is precisely this inherent dependence that makes us worry about the changed financial incentives under a regime like managed care (see e.g., Angell, 1993), where a physician's financial self-interest may be in conflict with the patient's need for care.

[27] The same dynamic holds in the research setting, usually with even greater force given the uncertainties of experimental environments. Every research protocol now gives great attention to designing appropriate consent forms and assuring uncoerced assent. But few believe that the average research subject is capable of evaluating fully the risks and benefits of his or her participation. Ultimately we rely on the ethics of researchers, and the oversight of Institutional Review Boards (human investigations committees), to assure that protocols' risks have been minimized and are reasonable given the knowledge expected. Here too we worry about conflicts of interest, where the roles of research investigator and care-giver are often conflated (Beauchamp and Childress, 1994).

[28] It is up to policy-makers, security specialists, system-implementers and health care practitioners to make sure that uninformed trust is not misplaced in matters related to IT. Individual informed consent will always be ethically important — a concrete expression

of our respect for autonomy. And, since economists have a faith that what happens at the margin controls all else, we can believe that the resistance of a few may serve to leverage considerable change. But "informed consent" to health data practice is more accurately expressive of social rather than individual acquiescence. That is, it is less about choice at the micro, patient-by-patient level (since so few can truly choose) and arguably more about appropriate, system-wide arrangements to which all will be subject. In the language of "social contracts," we must ask as philosophers do whether a hypothetical "reasonable person" from our society, fully apprised of the current state of information systems security and the risks attaching to information breaches, would consent to have his or her intimate medical information stored therein. Given what seem to be the manifest risks of the current environment, my own view is that a "yes" response is reasonable only on the assurance that we begin with established security models as a reference standard. Some reasonable burden of proof would then fall on practitioners and researchers to demonstrate that the health care system could not function without its own special rules, and that the probable benefits of any relaxation justified the risk.

[29] In the writings of political philosophers such as Locke (or the very different Hobbes or Rousseau), social contracts are the metaphorical mechanisms by which one assesses the desirability of arrangements that trade off individual rights to the community's needs. Without the community's protection, individual rights are completely insecure; so even die-hard individualists must be willing to yield a bit. Beyond the narrow confines of clinical care, the research and public health benefits of EMR systems are often generalized rather than individual, indeed even inter-generational. But these systemic benefits tend to flow precisely from practices that are the riskiest with respect to individual privacy, such as broad networking and aggregation of records for analysis. We are all potential experimental subjects now, given the uses to which our aggregated data may be put. We are all, also, part of an on-going experiment in the efficacy and safety of the IT systems in which our personal data will be stored.

[30] Is the protocol of this experiment "fair" to its subjects? It is too soon to say. But let us at least acknowledge what we do not know, try to curb both the Panglossian and Luddite rhetoric, and proceed at a pace appropriate to our ignorance. Information technology's great potential for both good and ill demands more careful analysis and less blind assertion than have traditionally obtained. Anyone who believes there will be easy, set-and-forget answers to the balance between individual and social goals — and the attendant parameters of health care information technology practice — is practicing a delusory, dangerous exceptionalism.

7. References

1. American Medical Association, *Code of Medical Ethics Current Opinions with Annotations* (Chicago IL: American Medical Association, 1994).
2. American Medical Record Association, "Position Paper on the Confidentiality of Medical Information," *Medical Record News* (December 1974).
3. Angell, Marcia, "The Doctor as Double Agent," *Kennedy Institute of Ethics Journal* 3 (1993): 279-286.
4. Arrow, Kenneth, J., "Uncertainty and the Welfare Economics of Medical Care," *American Economic Review* 53 (1963): 941-973.

5. Barrows, Randolph, and Clayton, Paul, "Privacy, Confidentiality and Electronic Medical Records," *Journal of the American Medical Informatics Association* 3 (1996): 139-148.
6. Beauchamp, Tom L., and Childress, James F., *Principles of Biomedical Ethics, Fourth Edition* (Oxford: Oxford University Press, 1994).
7. Blaug, Mark, *Economic Theory in Retrospect* (Cambridge UK: Cambridge University Press, 3rd edition, 1978)
8. Ernst & Young, *Third Annual Information Security Survey: Trends, Concerns and Practices* (New York NY: Ernst & Young, 1995a).
9. Ernst & Young, *Third Annual Information Security Survey: Trends, Concerns and Practices, A Focus on the Healthcare Industry* (New York NY: Ernst & Young, 1995b).
10. General Accounting Office, *Defense Achieves World-Wide Deployment of Composite Health Care System* (Washington DC: US Government Printing Office, 1996).
11. Gostin, Lawrence O., et al, "The Public Health Information Infrastructure: A National Review of the Law on Health Information Privacy,"*JAMA* 275 (26 June 1996): 1921-27.
12. Hiller, Marc. D. and Beyda, Vivian, "Computers, Medical Records and the Right to Privacy," *Journal of Health Politics, Policy and Law* 6 (Fall 1981): 463-487.
13. Institute of Medicine, *Modern Methods of Clinical Investigation* (Washington DC: National Academy Press, 1990).
14. Institute of Medicine, *The Computer-Based Patient Record: An Essential Technology for Health Care* (Washington DC: National Academy Press, 1991).
15. Institute of Medicine, *Health Data in the Information Age: Use, Disclosure and Privacy* (Washington, DC: National Academy, Press, 1994).
16. Joint Commission on the Accreditation of Hospitals, *Accreditation Manual for Hospitals* (Chicago IL: Joint Commission on the Accreditation of Hospitals, 1976).
17. National Research Council, *Information Technology in a Service Society* (Washington DC: National Academy Press, 1994).
18. Office of Technology Assessment, *Protecting Privacy in Computerized Medical Information* (Washington, DC: US Government Printing Office, 1993).
19. Office of Technology Assessment, *Identifying Health Technologies That Work: Searching for Evidence* (Washington DC: US Government Printing Office, 1994).
20. Office of Technology Assessment, *Issue Update on Information Security and Privacy in Network Environments* (Washington DC: US Government Printing Office, 1995)
21. Pauly, Mark V., "Is Medical Care Really Different?" in Warren Greenberg, Ed., *Competition in the Health Sector* (Germantown MD: Aspen Systems, 1978).
22. Regan, Priscilla M., *Legislating Privacy: Technology, Social Values, and Public Policy* (Chapel Hill: University of North Carolina Press, 1995).
23. Riley, John, "Open Secrets: Changes in Technology, Health Insurance Making Privacy a Thing of the Past." *Newsday,* 31 March 1996.
24. Schlesinger, Mark L. and Lee, T.K., "Is Health Care Different?" *Journal of Health Politics, Policy and Law* 18 (Fall 1993): 551-628.
25. Wald, Matthew, "Flight to Nowhere: Ambitious Update of Air Navigation Becomes a Fiasco," *New York Times*, 29 January 1996.

Clinical Record Systems in Oncology. Experiences and Developments on Cancer Registers in Eastern Germany

Bernd BLOBEL
The Otto-von-Guericke University Magdeburg, Faculty of Medicine, Institute of Biometrics and Medical Informatics, Leipziger Strasse 44, D-39120 Magdeburg, Germany

Abstract. Healthcare information systems have to guarantee quality and efficiency of the medical maintenance. The basis of such information systems is an good medical and caring documentation. The labour-shared, cooperative care for cancer patients as "Shared Care" requires a complete, distributed cancer documentation, summarized in clinical cancer registers. The information of those registers are also a basis for a population-related epidemiological registry. Cancer registers must meet all demands in data protection.

This paper deals with the security architecture of distributed information systems. Organizational as well as technical problems are discussed. Essential attention is paid to security modelling and access rights. The actual structure of the regional Clinical Cancer Register Magdeburg/Saxony-Anhalt and the existing as well as the planned register security mechanisms are presented.

1. Introduction

The healthcare system in the former GDR was characterized by a centralized organization structure. From the year 1989 [8], the following facts demonstrate the achievements, problems, and difficulties of healthcare. The expenditure for healthcare and social welfare increased up to 6.9% of the state budget, but also the healthcare suffered from the inefficiency economics, the objectively small resources, and the low technical standard. The inpatient care was realized in 543 hospitals with 165,950 beds. Providing outpatient care, 117 outpatient departments have been faced with 1,625 state doctor's practices, 2,024 doctor's medical services, 5,509 district nurse's stations, 1,327 nurse's medical services, and only 367 registred doctors. Nearly 600,000 employees worked for the healthcare. For each 10,000 inhabitants, the care was performed by 25.0 doctors, 7.8 dentists, and 2.6 pharmacists.

After the German reunification the healthcare and social welfare in Eastern Germany was adapted to the conditions in the "old" German Federal Republic. Accompanied by huge expenditures, this process will occupy yet a lot of years. The buildings have to be renovated, the equipment and the care structure must be brought up to date. The number of beds per hospitals was decreased and the number of registred doctors was increased extremely.

The reorganization of the healthcare system is directed towards an efficient healthcare system and medical informatics has to help realize this, as it will be shown in this paper.

2. The National Cancer Registry

All newly reported malignant neoplasms that occured in the former GDR have been recorded and entered into the „Nationales Krebsregister" (National Cancer Registry). This epidemiological register was one of the largest cancer registries of the world, founded in 1953. It was an population-based incidence register classified by place of residence. The cancer registration is based on the legal obligation of each doctor and dentist to declare all malignant neoplasms. Within a well developed cancer notification system, cancer control agencies for cancer patients were established in almost all of the more than 200 counties of the former GDR. Currently, the register includes detailed information of 2 million cancer patients, collected using an uniform questionnaire unchanged over the register's lifetime.

The major goals of the National Cancer Registry of the former GDR were

- the realization of medical statistics related to national cancer cases, supporting the decision-making by the State health authorities,
- the epidemiological research of malignant tumours.

The notification procedure ensures the recording of the tumor diagnosis, results of the first treatment, of additional measures, of follow-up and of autopsy in case of death. Each doctor or dentist was obliged by law to fill in a notification form and to transmit the form for evaluation to the National Cancer Registry through the local cancer control agencies performing quality assurance.

The registration was paper-based. For technical reasons in the eighthies only the centralized records were realized in a computerized manner.

The following details were recorded for each cancer case [27]:

- cancer patient's personal identification,
- tumour site,
- tumour histology, classified by the ICD-O,
- tumour stage,
- tumour diagnosis, related to the ICD9,
- tumour therapy,
- further treatment,
- follow up,
- individual anamnesis,
- family anamnesis,
- death, including autopsy results, if any.

These items correspond to sensitive personal and medical information.

The use of cancer documentation data was restricted and audited. Besides rules for the confidential doctor-patient relationship there were no security measures like encoding of records etc. From the technical point of view the National Cancer Registry was a closed system.

After the German reunification some cases of security offences, e.g. related to special patients' medical record, were announced, perpetrated in the GDR healthcare by the state security service. Such misdemeanours in relation to the cancer registry the author cannot verify, but also not exclude. Apart from dissidents or similarly evaluated persons, there were practically no social or related threats for patients within the GDR society, concerning e.g. the revelation of medical information by insurance companies or others.

About 99% of the malignant neoplasms were registered in the National Cancer Registry. Only <1% was recorded by death certificates only (DCO). Initially there were political restrictions for work with and interpretation of the information concerned with the cancer register, but also technical problems hindered the successful use of that excellent scientific source.

In the former Federal Republic of Germany such registry was not available. Only the Saarland has created a comparable institution. After the German reunification the legal basis for the continuation of the National Cancer Registry was missing. Big efforts had to be made, to save the National Cancer Registry from extermination. First, the registry was adopted by the 5 "new" German Federal States and Berlin with an administrative agreement. By a quickly elaborated and passed law for saving the cancer register („Krebsregistersicherungsgesetz“ [6]) the continuation of registration and the restricted use of the cancer data for research was made possible until the December 31th, 1994. Since January 1st, 1995, the Cancer Registry Law („Krebsregistergesetz“) is legally valid, after having been discussed for more than 10 years and finally accelerated by the circumstances and legal problems with the National Cancer Registry [7].

The procedure of the population-based cancer registration is realized in two steps by two institutions. In the first stage, the Trusted Site accumulates the patient-related tumour data recorded by doctors, dentists, Follow-up Organization Centres or Clinical Cancer Registers (see later). Only few items about the cancer case, needed for a population-related cancer incidence register are recorded. The Trusted Site anonymizes the cancer patient's personal data by an asymmetric procedure, e.g. a hybrid IDEA-RSA encoding. The identifying data will be encoded with an IDEA session key, generated accidentally. The IDEA key will be encoded by a public RSA key with a minimal length of 640 bit. To allow an unambiguous assigning of additional information to the correct patient record, a control number (a special kind of pseudonyms) will be generated, using different attributes of the personal data. That control number will be generated by the utilization of a one-way procedure (MD5) and a symmetrically cryptographic algorithm (IDEA). To allow the assigning of data from the different federal states, the control number procedure and key have to be united Germany-wide ("Linkage Format"). The Trusted Site transfers both the encoded patient-identifying data and the epidemiological plaintext data to the Registry Site. The Registry Site stores the record in the register database and brings together different registrations belonging to one patient. After the matching of data, an accidental number will be added to the control number and the result will be symmetrically encoded by IDEA ("Storage Format"). For the record linkage, the control numbers must be transformed from the "Storage Format" to the "Linkage Format". A corresponding security infrastructure (TTP services like key management) is necessary.

On request, the exploitation of anonymized register data is possible for scientific aims, restricted in time and number. In special medical cases a trustworthy advisory committee can also authorize the use of reidentified records. The procedure applied in the context of the epidemiological cancer registry was developed by *Appelrath* and *Michaelis* [11, 26].

In the context of reorganization and reformation of the Eastern Germany's healthcare system and his adaption to the Western Germany's conditions, there was a big chance to design the healthcare system with the latest technology and according to the actual requirements in industrial countries all over the world.

3. Background Conditions in Healthcare

The basic conditions of the future healthcare systems in the industrialized countries are characterized

- by the demographic development with an increasing number of multimorbid persons,
- by the rapid medical and technical progress as well as
- by increasing demands on the quality of life also regarding disease and suffering, disabilities and chronic diseases.

Taking these basic conditions into account, the industrial countries are trying to realize an efficient healthcare within the health policy framework [19], which is determined objectively as well as subjectively. The efficiency of healthcare must be evaluated by both the managerial and the economical efficiency (cost-benefit relation, outcome) **but also** by the quality of medical outcome. Regarding this

- specialization and shared labour in both healthcare and welfare as "Shared Care",
- communication and cooperation between the care givers, but also between providers and funding organizations, e.g. insurance companies, and/or other institutions directly or indirectly involved in healthcare as well as
- competition on the basis of corresponding transparency of achievements and flexibility

must be developed [19]. These processes are accompanied by an improvement in technology in health institutions, especially in information technology.

Traditionally, information systems support achievement-related (outcome-related) evaluation and compensation as well as an optimal interoperability between the different healthcare providers. The outcome evaluation is required for the ascertainment of an achievement-related reimbursement as well as for a corresponding transparency of costs and achievements. Internally such transparency is useful for an optimal arrangement and management of the processes. Externally it serves the productivity certificate facing the potential partners in cooperation or facing the funding organizations. Increasingly, the medical objectives, i.e. the direct care processes and their optimization, will become dominant. The information systems meeting these requirements must be established nearly real-time and process-oriented as well as patient-centred. The system architecture has to be designed according to the complex model of the real processes. Such an information system architecture is very demanding with respect to data security.

Also the care of cancer patients should be organized in an efficient manner. A specialized and labour-shared cancer care as well as a secure distributed tumour documentation meet these requirements.

4. Structure of Hospital Information Systems

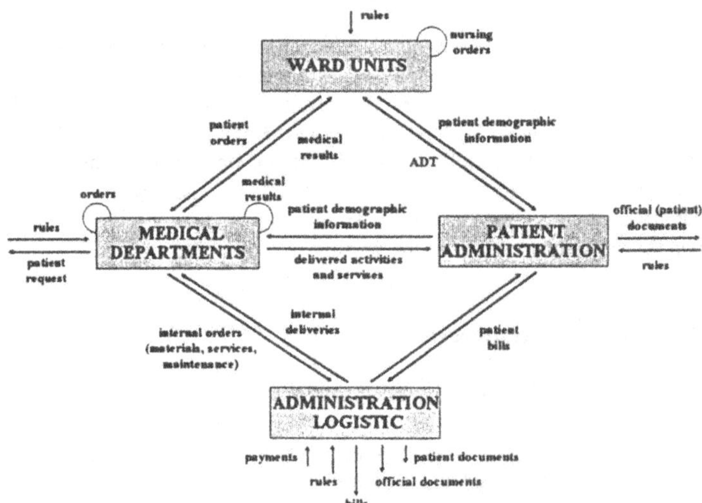

Figure 1: General model of a Hospital Information System

The architecture of information systems corresponding to the described demands should be explained using the example of Hospital Information Systems (HIS) [4]. Figure 1 shows the streams of information and materials within a hospital as well as between hospital and its associated area (modified according to [1]). The representation formalizes the actual processes of labour-shared medical care within a hospital. If the general HIS model will be realized by actual application systems which are distributed in analogy to the underlying processes, this can be illustrated as shown in figure 2.

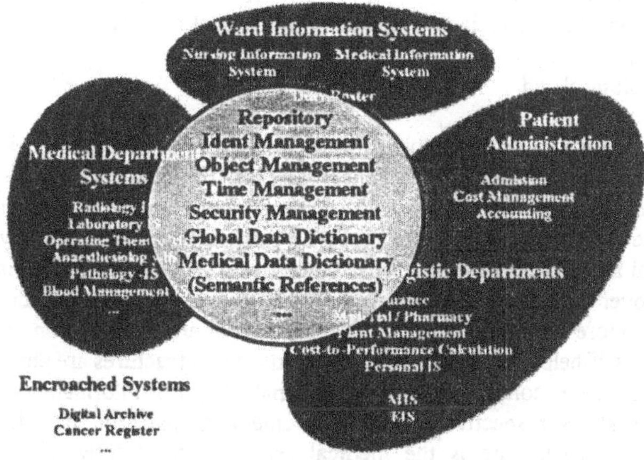

Figure 2: HIS characterized by applications

5. General System Structure

The systems associated with the individual work fields must copy and support the actual care process optimally by information. They must communicate or still better cooperate like in the real labour-sharing world. To guarantee a semantically determined communication and cooperation, different logically "centralized" functions are necessary. This includes extended identification management, object management ("Extended Object Directory") with indexation, time management for the supply of ressources without conflicts, security management, a global "Data Dictionary" for the navigation between (preferably database-based) applications, a medical "Data Dictionary" for the semantic reference as well as a complex "Repository".

These logical "centralized" functions will be realized in the HANSA project [1] for open, distributed, modular, networked healthcare information systems. Among other things [21], it deals with the "Identification and Authentication Manager", with the "Rule Manager", and with the "Security Manager". which will be processed by the Magdeburg team.

[1] The HANSA project (Healthcare Advanced Networked System Architecture) is funded by the European Commission within the fourth framework "Telematics Applications Programmme". It is coordinated by *Frabrizio Massimo Ferrara* (Rome).

6. Definition of "Shared Care"

Corresponding to [20] the "Shared Care" can be defined as
"a continuous and coordinated activity of
different persons in
different institutions under
employment of different methods at
different times
in order to be able to help patients optimally with respect to their
medical,
psychological and
social being".

The cancer care is a vivid example of the "Shared Care" concept in healthcare. From the first suspicion or ascertainment of a cancer disease, the diagnostics follows in specialized institutions (usually in hospitals, but also in special ambulances or in specialist's practices). Currently, the therapy is likewise accomplished in specialized sites (usually in hospitals, but also in special ambulances or in specialist's practices). However, also an increasing number of GPs take over these tasks themselves and/or at least organize or coordinate the care. The same is true more than ever for the follow up, where, in addition, also rehabilitation organizations, self-help groups and other "Shared Care" structures are entering.

The "Shared Care" concept requires an optimal design of informational relationships and information systems respectively. The convenient system for the documentation and information in medical care is the medical record. Consistently, a process-related and patient-centred information system dominated by medical and caring aspects is realized by an electronic patient record (EPR, electronic medical record, computerized patient record, ...) [19, 29]. Within healthcare delivery structures, which are organized labour-shared and distributed, the electronic patient record is the way to support the care.

For the support of area-covering evenly high-degree care of cancer patients, so called cancer centres or oncological centres were founded in Germany. With generous funding through the German Federal Ministry of Health, a network of about 20 such institutions was installed also in Eastern Germany [3, 4]. Apart from clinical cancer registers, epidemiological cancer registers are also very helpful for the investigation of some cancer-related questions, as mentioned in paragraph 2. In 1993, the "new" German federal countries and Berlin have decided to continue the common epidemiological cancer registration in Berlin, called „Gemeinsames Krebsregister“. The clinical cancer registers are the dominant registration sites for the data flow to this Berlin registry. Following, I will restrict my presentation mainly to the regional Clinical Cancer Register Magdeburg/Saxony-Anhalt.

Within the cancer centres, which were founded

- to support the cooperation between the different institutions relating to the labour-shared care of cancer patients,
- to improve quality and efficiency of cancer care,
- to promote research and development in oncology,
- to improve training and education,
- to elaborate standards for care and quality assurance etc.,

the clinical cancer registers should support the authorized user to achieve these objectives by available, integer and consistent information at the right time and at the right place.

Logically, the regional Clinical Cancer Register Magdeburg/Saxony-Anhalt supports the "Shared Care" concept in Oncology.

7. The Legal Framework of Cancer Registers

The arrangement of processes in a society and therefore also in healthcare is bound to the legal framework, to professional regulations as well as to institutional instructions and guidelines. But especially in medicine, ethical criterias, psychological conditions and social consequences must be considered [15, 16, 23, 24].

The legal basis for the function of cancer registers are

- the general legislation of documentation in medicine,
- the regulations of the „Bundesdatenschutzgesetz" (the federal data protection law) as well as the „Landesdatenschutzgesetze" (the data protection laws of the different federal states),
- professional regulations for physicians, nurses and equivalent professionals in relation to medical processes and medical data (e.g. the obligation of secrecy),
- the orders of the criminal law.

Within the European Union, the EU Data Protection Directive, passed by the Council of Europe in the summer 1995, is also an attractive legal basis. But the transformation into the German legislation is rather unlikely due to the principle of subsidiarity [5].

Amongst all, the special legal framework for the function of epidemiological cancer registers are established in the already cited German Cancer Registry Law [7]. These general regulations will be specified by corresponding „Landes-Krebsregistergesetze" (cancer register laws of the different German federal states), which will be extended to some instructions on clinical cancer registers.

The medical documentation and especially cancer registers must be carried out in such a way, that the patient's right of informational self-determination is guaranteed and that hygenic, mental, social harm or even existential threats are kept away. But there are also objective aspects and constraints, determining record, storage and processing of patient information. Such aspects and constraints are in patient's interest or absolutely necessary for the staging of medical care. In this context the civil rights of health professionals, which are defined in professional regulations or in the works constitution law for employed health professionals, are also noteworthy. Security measures in medicine should also improve the common legal security.

A basic condition of recording, processing and communication of personal data is in general the consent of the concerned, but at least his/her information. For implementation of patient-related documentation and information systems the three dimensions of security have always to be guaranteed [12]; i.e.

- integrity
- availability and
- confidentiality.

Currently the legal basis of recording, processing and communication of patient related oncological data is the patient consent.

8. The Security Background in the Magdeburg Department of Medical Informatics

The Magdeburg department is the medical informatics group with the most extended activities and experiences on data security in modern information systems in Germany. In 1993 the first hardware based solution for trusted communication in the German healthcare was implemented in the Clinical Cancer Register Magdeburg/Saxony-Anhalt. The research and development as well as the implementation of security measures in productive medical information systems is realized in two organizational and technological phases. In the first phase, we have implemented secure communication and interoperability between different institutions, assumed as closed systems. Following, we have installed a secure external communication infrastructure. Within the organizations therefore, we have guaranteed traditional measures, like organizational instructions and rules, physical measures in the departments, password systems, audit, network security mechanisms etc. The internal infrastructure was considered secure. The second phase is characterized by trusted communication and cooperation in an insecure world. The challenge of such strategy is to overcome the implementation of security measure in both client and server systems. In this context we are currently incorporated into different projects, funded by the European Commission in the fourth framework "Telematic Applications Programme". The activities are addressed to the different views of security in medical informatics

- as the definition of general objectives and conditions and as the management of processes and measures [2],
- the development of security utilities, facilities, and services in modern healthcare information system architectures [3],
- the development, realization, and evaluation of trusted communication by secure authentication and Trusted Third Party services [4],
- the realization and evaluation of all these features in the context of some special applications in realistic healthcare environment, like "Shared Care", network based as well as chip card based heterogeneous information system architecture [5].

Therefore, the Magdeburg Department of Medical Informatics performs activities on all relevant topics of complex data security in medicine, demonstrated in a typical example of labour-shared and regional organized care.

9. General Guidelines for Development and Implementing of a Secure Clinical Cancer Register

In 1990/1991, we have started the development and implementation of an integrated hospital information system (HIS) at the Magdeburg University Hospital. Since then we have to realize all activities, covering the systems development, like specification, design, realization and testing of components of our HIS. The developed components have to be integrated in an existing organizational, functional and technical environment for production.

Since the introducing of IT-applications must be oriented on the objectives and processes of the concerned institution, the most important activity is a clear and complete description of the enterprice policy (objectives; measures; management, process and quality criterias). The second activity should deal with complex process analysis, including integration mechanisms. Then a general risk analysis of the system environment as well as the definition of threats and countermeasures have to be performed. Quality management and system evaluation as development results are often unsatisfactory, nevertheless they are essential.

---

[2]These activities run in the ISHTAR project (Implementation of Secure Healthcare Telematics Applications in Europe; coordinator: *Barry Barber*, Birmingham) as a part of the fourth framework "Telematics Applications Programme", sponsored by the European Commission under use of the results of the SEISMED project of the third EC framework "Advanced Informatics in Medicine (AIM)".

[3] These activities are running in the HANSA project.

[4]These works are accomplished within the TRUSTHEALTH1 project (Trustworthy Health Telematics) as part ot the fourth framework "Telematics Applications Programmme", sponsored by the European Commission. The project is coordinated altogether by *Gunnar Klein* (SPRI Stockholm) and nationally by *Otto Rienhoff* (Göttingen).

[5]DIABCARD projects as parts of the third and/or. the fourth framework of the European commission (coordinator: *Rolf Engelbrecht*, Munich).

A general prerequisite is a clear description of the responsibilities within the institution as well as in the supplier enterprice. We have good experiences with the appointment of a General Manager (preferably a specialist in organizational and IT issues) in the person of the Medical Informatics Department's head and with specialized responsibilities for each activity and topic respectively. In Germany the involvement of the works committee is subject to legislation. But also in countries without such regulations, such involvement should be done as early as possible, for instance by the inclusion of the concerned personnel. All activities must be documented and in the performing phase protocolled in detail.

For each step, the continuous propagation of high level security policy, the improvement of security awareness, and also the training and education of the management as well as the employees is very important. These aspects had always our special attention. It proved difficult, that the Medical Informatics staff could develop the whole concept, but that the components were realized both by ourselves and by external suppliers. That means, that the philosophy must be adopted to the different development environments and possibilities of the supplier in a compromizing sense, but preserving some basic principles.

In order that information systems are approximately as close to reality as possible, the different applications must be able to cooperate. To bring about cooperativity or interoperability of subsystems, the system has to realize the integration type "Integration" [17]. However this implicates that all functions and methods are defined at the database level. Only object-oriented databases have overcome this challenge.

We took the decision for INGRES as the application system database and the development environment. The choice was founded on the property of INGRES as the first relational DB to realize object-oriented features like the knowledge base, rule, trigger events and stored procedures. Meanwhile all dominant DBs have implemented such functions and possibilities and we have installed applications, based on different wide-spread databases, like Oracle, Informix, Sybase and so on.

10. General Security Architectures

The general architecture of distributed cooperating information systems is demonstrated in figure 3. The first requirement is to guarantee the communication of legitimated personnel in a trusted manner only. For this reason a corresponding security infrastructure must be established. In the following chapters this complex of trustworthy communication is described as communication security.

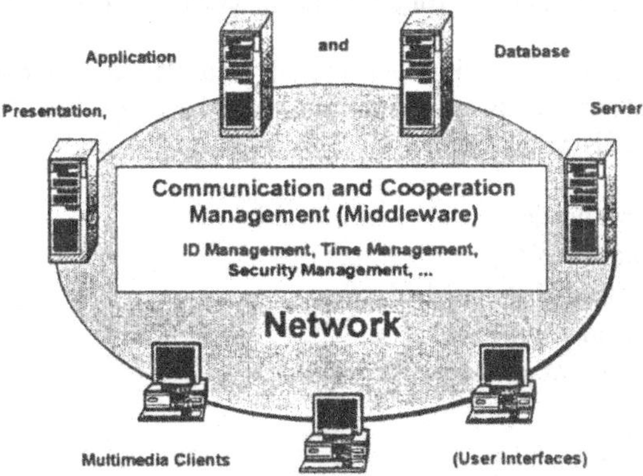

Figure 3: General architecture of distributed cooperating information systems

The authorities within the security infrastructure have to be trustees by their structure as well as in the authority's legal relation to the communication partners and their interests. This is the only way, by which the authorities as references can guarantee trustworth.
The main task of the security infrastructure in respect to the communication security is the provable guarantee of the communication partners' authentication amongst themselves as well as towards third persons or organizations. For this function and for the protection of information integrity one is using certified electronic signatures.

Another important prerequisite for the communication of medical (that means in general highly sensitive) data is the confidentiality of communication, which must work between the partners in the sense of addressed confidentiality without any functional or other restrictions (e.g. performance). Such confidentiality of the contents of information is realized by using cryptographic measures. Symmetric as well as asymmetric algorithms are implemented.

The second requirement for security architectures deals with the functional and data access restrictions for legitimated personnel. In the following chapters this complex of restricted functional as well as data access rigths is described as application security. The basis for application security management is the different position and function of the personnel within the healthcare. Especially, in this context the doctor-patient-relationship, privacy and confidentiality as well as the real process of medical treatment and care are essential.

11. Required Infrastructure for Communication Security

As pronounced, the installation of secure communication systems requires a security infrastructure, which is realized by trustworthy authorities in form of *T*rusted *T*hird *P*arty (TTP) services. Functions of the security infrastructure (TTP services) are for instance

- the generation, distribution and management of keys,
- the promotion and maintenance of name services (directories),
- the certification of keys,
- the time services (certified timestamps) and
- other notary's office functions.

Within a German model project for using health professional cards (HPC) [6] as a part of the TRUSTHEALTH project, we are preparing the development and implementation of the corresponding security infrastructure in the environment of the Clinical Cancer Register Magdeburg/Saxony-Anhalt. In this context it was remarkable, that not only natural persons (individuals), but also legal persons (organizations) should be able to communicate in a secure manner.

For the use of HPC as electronic identity cards and also as electronically vocational identification, the following trustworthy structure must be established. As a result of the German TRUSTHEALTH project group [10], we plan for the German model project the following authorities:

- for the personal authentication
  - the Naming Authority (NA),
    resulting in a personal distinguished name
  - the Registration Authority (RA),
    resulting in an authentic personal document

[6] This German model project of the „Arbeitsgemeinschaft Karten im Gesundheitswesen" is chaired by Otto Rienhoff (Goettingen) and includes also the HPC-use in an intensive care ward of the Goettingen University Hospital [2].

- for the professional authentication
  - the Qualification Authentication Authority (QAA), *resulting in a qualification authentication*
  - the Profession Authentication Authority (PAA), *resulting in a profession authentication*
  - the Professional Registration Authority (PRA), *resulting in an authentic professional document*
- for the professional certification
  - the Professional Certification Authority (PCA),
- for the professional class authentication
  - the Professional Class Definer (PCD) *resulting in a professional class definition*
  - the Professional Naming Authority (PNA), *resulting in a professional class distinguished name*
  - the Professional Class Registration Authority (PCRA), *resulting in an authentic professional class document*
- for the key certification
  - the Key Generation Instance (KGI) *resulting in a public (and a privat) key* *resulting in a public (and a privat) class key*
  - the Certification Authority (CA) *resulting in a public key certificate*

There is a common consideration of identity and profession within the context of the application in the case of cancer registers. Therefore, a general authority (C)A could be useful, which also certificates the keys. For general purposes chip cards, the separation of the CA for both the identity and the profession should be recommended. Figure 4 presents the planned structure of security infrastructure authorities in the regional cancer register.

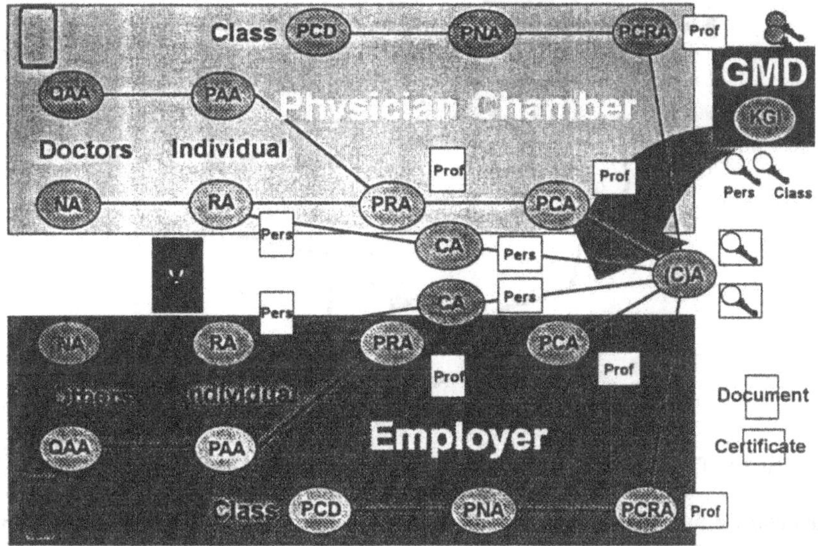

Figure 4: The planned structure of security infrastructure authorities

12. The Security Architecture of the Regional Clinical Cancer Register Magdeburg/Saxony-Anhalt

The foundation and further development of the Clinical Cancer Register Magdeburg/Saxony-Anhalt in 1992/1993 was persecuted to realize a regionally distributed EPR in Oncology, which is usable for all institutions and individuals, labour-shared involved in the cancer care. This pioneer achievement could only be realized with pioneer achievements on the data security domain. Therefore, the Magdeburg cancer register was the first medical institution in Germany, designing and realizing data security in medicine systematically. On account of our objectives, additional to the cancer register functions [19], the functionality of intra-institutional and inter-institutional communication by online-documentation as well as online-information has been forced.

Currently, 53 clinics of the Magdeburg University Hospital and of other important hospitals in the governmental district Magdeburg are involved in the regional cancer register. To establish the register as a continuous and patient-centred cancer documentation, the crucial breakthrough could be achieved with the integration of the Oncological Follow up Organization Centre for registered doctors into our cancer register. By the direct and secure connection of the Follow up Organization Centre LAN to the GTDS, also the GP's Follow up structures (registered doctors) could be involved into the syntactically and semantically unified form of documentation and information. In this context, the Oncological Follow up Organization Centre realizes both the function of a documentation place and the institution for follow up organization in mission of registered doctors (GPs). Figure 5 gives an overview of the geographic structure of the Clinical Cancer Register Magdeburg/Saxony-Anhalt. The catchment area of the register includes the north of our federal country (with a total 2.8 million inhabitants) with about 1.2 millions inhabitants.

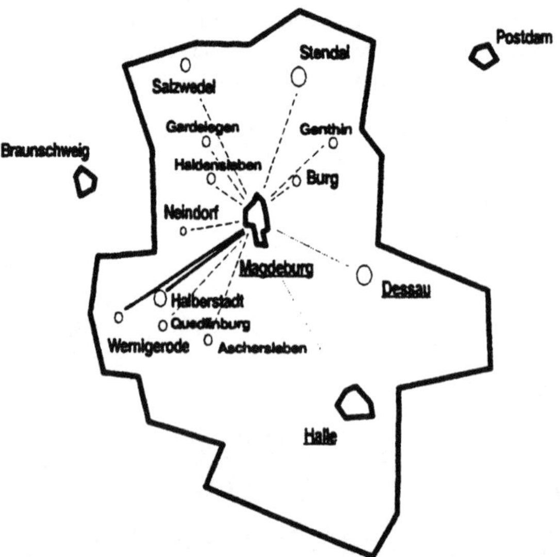

Figure 5: The catchment area of the Magdeburg/Saxony-Anhalt Cancer Register

An optimal effect of the documentation and information system is only achievable with an online connection of all participants. This means, that the system has to be integrated into the oncological care like a realtime system. Currently about one fourth of the partners are working online with the GTDS. At the end of next year all partners will cooperate online with our register.

The regional cancer register contains the patient-related general tumor medical records for all institutions and/or persons, which are integrated in the register and are included into the labour-shared care of cancer patients. As pronounced, the cancer documentation is realized on the basis of the voluntary, written consent of the informed patient with respect to the cooperative tumor documentation. Restraints of the documentation, desired by the patient, e.g. the exclusion of individual persons or institutions from the communication combine, can be realized. However, that must remain the exception, because otherwise the objective of the project would be put in question. Since the general cancer record is a collection of personal, highly sensitive data, particular measures guaranteeing data protection and data security had to be realized. These data security measures concern

- measures in the local networks of the respective user departments, e.g.
  - the design of a communication network structure with attention to legal and managerial (structural, organizational) significance,
  - the implementation of all server equipments as security areas (DB server; application server; communication server, like router, HL7 server etc.; transaction monitors, authority server etc.),
  - security mechanisms of the LAN, like access nodes, address lists, special gateways for external communication (modem, fax, BTX) as well as KAPI (or better S-KAPI) protocols for ISDN communication (see for details [16]),
- measures for the communication by the public telephone system
  - analogous lines, ISDN,

  and/or
- other communication media of third parties
  - e.g. the scheduled Magdeburg Metropolitan Area Network (MAN), the German scientific information network (WIN) of the DFN union as an example of a Wide Area Network (WAN)).

On one hand, the guarantee of data security includes organizational measures. Among others, the following points are relevant:

- the restraint of the user domains and authorized users to the necessary extension,
- the definition of user groups and the respective rights (functional and data access rights) of these groups,
- a four level identification and authentication system and an extended audit.

Apart from that, organizational and technical measures were realized, such as the exclusive use of the cancer register server for the tumor documentation application as well as the separation of the production mode system from the test & development & training system. Through such measures, the unauthorized access to the application by persons authorized to system access can be prevented. In the same context, the control of the functional and the access rights was realized by the network architecture (communication units and routers). Additionally, an extended password-related access control should be at least realized.

In the first phase of the implementation and the productive work of the regional cancer register, no secure hardware-based identification and authentication including the corresponding right management of individual users was available apart from the three-stage password mechanism and the log-file system. Therefore, an architecture of distributed, closed and secure external subsystems was realized first. The identification and authentication of area and/or client (system) and consequently the access control was realized for the external users connected by analogous lines and modems on the basis of MACS (Modem Access Control System, FAST company). For external users, connected by ISDN, we have installed the Kryptogard LAN L3 equipment (Kryptocom company). This system realizes a secure LAN-to-LAN communication, including firewall functionalities. The information encoding is performed by the application of Triple-DES session keys. These keys are exchanged with RSA encryption, on this way ensuring both the identification and authentication of the coupled domain and the integrity check of communication. Meanwhile also the secure installation of single PC by ISDN Kryptogard PC (Kryptocom company) could be implemented. Figure 6 presents the successful temporary solution in the topicality of May 1996.

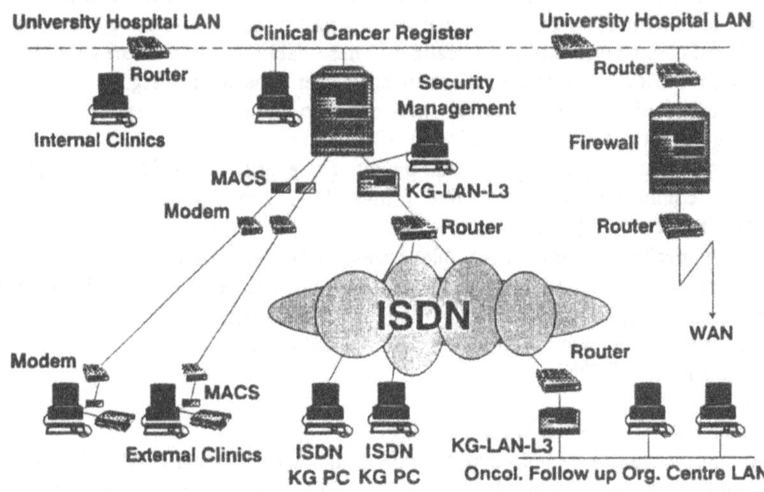

Figure 6: Productive security solution in the regional distributed cancer register

In this context, two development activities should be remembered

- the identification and authentication on the basis of Trusted Third Party services and health professional cards within both the TRUSTHEALTH and the cited German model project,
- a detailed right management (security management of the specific application-related functional and data access rights) in the DHE-framework (Distributed Healthcare Environment) of the HANSA project.

The functional and data access rights result on the one hand from the structural and organizational conditions (classification of users, user hierarchy), and on the other hand from the actual care process (doctor in charge of the case, the confidential doctor-patient relationship, temporary diagnostic and/or therapeutic team). The structural determined right management can be described by Mandatory Access Models (extended matrix of access rights). The patient-related right management has to be described by Discretionary Access Models. In order to master the system, groups and rules for users and rights respectively are defined, which are to be examined for the concrete case. The modelling of the security management based on a defined security policy [7] is discussed [17]. If available, the transfer

[7] These activities run in the ISHTAR project (Implementation of Secure Healthcare Telematics Applications in Europe; coordinator: *Barry Barber*, Birmingham) as a part of the fourth framework "Telematics Applications Programme", sponsored by the European Commission under use of the results of the SEISMED project of the third EC framework "Advanced Informatics in Medicine (AIM)".

and the storage of data should be implemented in a cryptographically encoded form. Figure 7 represents the general scheme of security systems, while figure 8 demonstrates security services in multi-stage client-server architectures.

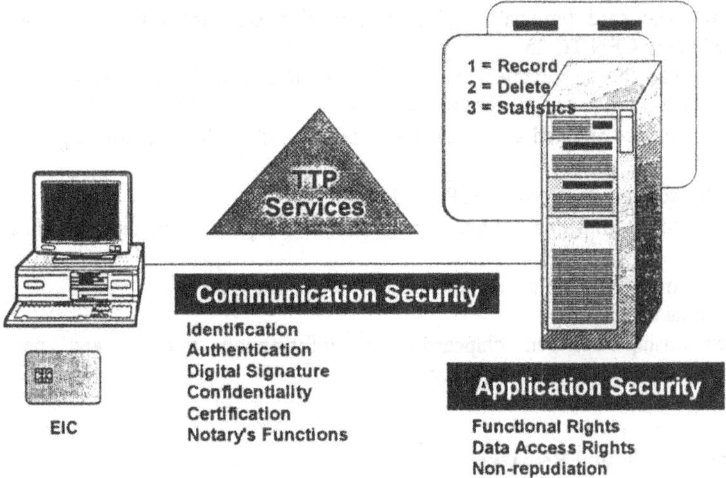

Figure 7: General scheme of security systems

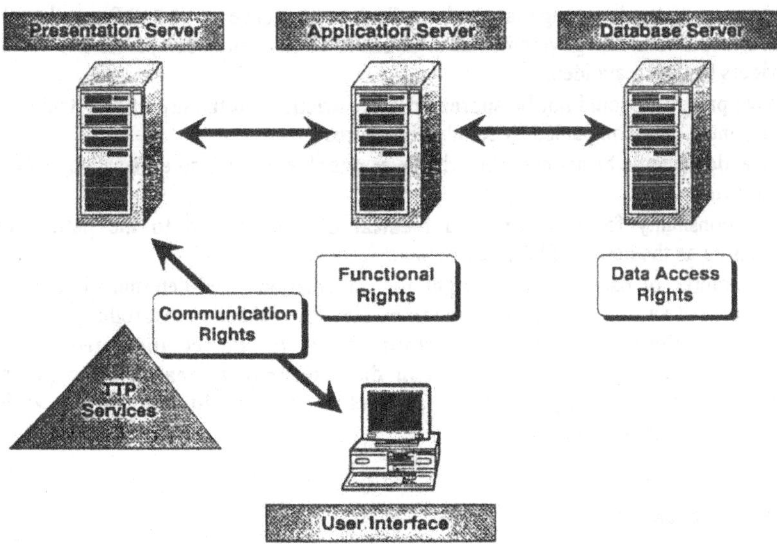

Figure 8: Security services in multi-stage client-server architectures

The success of security measures depends on the security awareness of all related persons, which requires extended education and training.

For the pilot project of the regional Clinical Cancer Register Magdeburg/Saxony-Anhalt the complete furnishing of all partners with HPC and card readers is planned for 1997. That means the installation of about 300 HPC and 200 card readers. As in the pilot's first phase, the card reader will correspond to the „Multifunktionales Kartenterminal"-Standard (MKT, multi-functional card terminal) [1]. Currently, this standard for a T=1 card reader is discussed in the CEN TC 251.

To standardize the development and implementation activities as well as to improve the quality of work, the use of modern tools, like

- tools for object-oriented system analysis, design and implementation (e.g. SOM, SERM) [28],
- tools for security analysis (SIDERO) [22],
- the SEISMED guidelines with the comprehensive expert's experience and knowledge [9, 13, 14],
- and own modelling and development tools for secure systems

is an essential basis.

The relationship between chipcard-based information systems and network-based information systems is discussed in e.g. [19, 25].

13. Some Concluding Remarks

- Medical care, care providers' outcome and personal data security are not contradictionally but conditionally.
- Legal conditions, issues, involved persons, requirements and goals as well as need of protection are especially important for planning and performing of health data communication.
- The merge of legal, managerial, and medical competence of the different healthcare-related institutions like governmental organizations, insurance companies and healthcare providers has to be avoided.
- Medical progress should not be supressed by restrictions in the use of new technologies, but this must be accompanied by suitable measures.
- Medical data should be anonymized whenever possible, using also especial algorithms like pseudonyms.
- The responsibility for patient-related medical data is located to the patient-doctor-relationship as the kernel of healthcare.
- The guarantee of patient's human right for informational self-determination requires a higher level of awareness and education to be able for realization that right.

The general higher threats for persons have to be compensated by legal, organizational, and technical measures in data security to realize ethic principles, professional's responsibility and the protection of the human rights within a democratic and liberal society.

14. Acknowledgement

The author is obliged to the European Commission, DG XIII, to the SEISMED Consortium and to the other EU projects for the support of the activities as well as to the Ministry of Education and Sciences of the Federal State of Saxony-Anhalt for funding.

References

[1] Arbeitsgemeinschaft „Karten im Gesundheitswesen", GMD - Forschungszentrum Informationstechnik GmbH: Multifunktionale KartenTerminals (MKT) für das Gesundheitswesen und andere Anwendungsgebiete. Spezifikation Version 0.9, August 1995.

[2] Arbeitskreis „Health Professional Card" der Arbeitsgemeinschaft „Karten im Gesundheitswesen": Deutscher Modellversuch „Health Professional Card (HPC)", Göttingen, 13.3.1996.

[3] Bundesministerium für Gesundheit: Anforderungen für Modellvorhaben zur Verbesserung der regionalen onkologischen Zusammenarbeit. Bonn, 13.6.1991.

[4] Bundesministerium für Gesundheit: Grundsätze für den Aufbau und Betrieb Klinischer Krebsregister in Behandlungsschwerpunkten zur flächendeckenden regionalen onkologischen Versorgung. Bonn, 17.6.1991.

[5] Council of Europe: EU Directive on the Protection of Individuals with Regard to the Processing of Personal Data and on the Free Movement of such Data. Strassbourg 1995.

[6] Gesetz zur Sicherung und vorläufigen Fortführung der Datensammlung des „Nationalen Krebsregisters" der ehemaligen Deutschen Demokratischen Republik (Krebsregistersicherungsgesetz) vom 29.12.1992, BGBl I, 2335.

[7] Gesetz über Krebsregister (Krebsregistergesetz, -KRG) vom 4.11.1994, BGBl I, 3351.

[8] Institut für Medizinische Statistik und Datenverarbeitung Berlin (Hrsg.): Das Gesundheitswesen der Deutschen Demokratischen Republik 1989. 24. Jahrgang, Berlin 1989.

[9] SEISMED Consortium: European Health Data Security Guidelines. IT and Security Personnel. Birmingham 1995.

[10] TRUSTHEALTH1 Consortium - German Group: German Recommendations to the TTP Functional Specification (Draft). Göttingen 1996.

[11] H.-J. Appelrath, J. Michaelis, I. Schmidtmann, W. Thoben: Empfehlung an die Bundesländer zur technischen Umsetzung der Verfahrensweise gemäß Gesetz über Krebsregister (KRG). Technischer Bericht, Tumorzentrum Rheinland-Pfalz, Mainz 1995.

[12] A.R. Bakker: Security in Medical Information Systems. In: J.H. van Bemmel and A.T. McCray (Edrs.): Yearbook of Medical Informatics, pp 52-60. Schattauer, Stuttgart 1993.

[13] B. Barber, J. Davey: The Use of the CCTA Risk Analysis and Management Methodology [CRAMM] in Health Information Systems. In: K.C. Lun, P. Degoulet, T.E. Piemme, O. Rienhoff (Edrs.): MEDINFO 92, pp. 1589-1593. North Holland, Amsterdam 1992.

[14] B. Barber, G. Bleumer, J. Davey, K. Louwerse: How to Achieve Secure Environments for Information Systems in Medicine. In: R.A. Greenes, H.E. Peterson, D.J. Protti (Edrs.): MEDINFO 96, pp. 635-639. North Holland, Amsterdam 1996.

[15] B. Blobel: Datensicherheitsprobleme und -lösungen in offenen medizinischen Informationssystemen. In: B. Blobel (Hrsg.): Datenschutz in medizinischen Informationssystemen, S. 123-138. Verlag Vieweg, Braunschweig - Wiesbaden 1995.

[16] B. Blobel: Open Information Systems and Data Security in Medicine. In: B. Barber, A. Treacher and K. Louwerse (Edrs.): Towards Security in Medical Telematics, pp 168-182. IOS Press, Amsterdam - Oxford - Tokyo - Washington/DC 1996.

[17] B. Blobel: Modelling for Design and Implementation of Secure Health Information Systems. In: A. R. Bakker et al. (Edrs.): Communicating Health Information in an Insecure World. Conference Preprint, pp 149-156. Data Protection and Security Working Conference, Helsinki 30 September - 3 October 1995.

[18] B. Blobel: Konzeption für Telematikanwendungen im Gesundheitswesen sowie für ältere und behinderte Menschen. Zuarbeit zum Entwurf des Durchführungskonzeptes für eine Telematik-Initiative Sachsen-Anhalt. Magdeburg, 19. Februar 1996.

[19] B. Blobel: A Regional, Secure Cancer Documentation System for an Optimal "Shared Care" in Oncology. Presentation at the MIE '96, Copenhagen, August 1996.

[20] K.-H. Ellsässer, C. O. Köhler: Shared Care: Konzept einer verteilten Pflege - Kurz- und langfristige Perspektiven in Europa. Informatik, Biometrie und Epidemiologie in Medizin und Biologie 24 (1993) H.4, S. 188-198.

[21] F.M. Ferrara: The EDITH Approach: The Management Of Authorization And Security In Healthcare Information Systems. In: B. Barber, A Treacher and K. Louwerse (Edrs.): Toward Security in Medical Telematics - Legal and Technical Aspects, pp 200-213. IOS Press, Amsterdam - Oxford - Tokyo - Washington/DC 1996.

[22] E. Flikkenschild, P.v.d. Sluijs, E. Buis, J. Verhage: SIDERO: a relational Database Application for Security Practitioners, supporting the implementation of SEISMED guidelines in Health Care Institutions. AIM SEISMED Deliverable. Leiden 1996.

[23] E.-H.W. Kluge: Health Information, Privacy, Confidentiality and Ethics. B. Barber, A.R. Bakker, S. Bengtson (Edrs.): Caring for Health Information Safety, Security and Secrecy, pp. . Elsevier, Amsterdam 1994.

[24] E.-H.W. Kluge: Health information, the fair information principles and ethics. In: J.H. van Bemmel and A.T. McCray (Edrs.): Yearbook of Medical Informatics, pp 255-264. Schattauer, Stuttgart 1995.

[25] C.O. Köhler, W. Schuster: Informationelle Selbstbestimmung des Patienten durch die Patientenkarte. In: B. Blobel (Hrsg.): Datenschutz in medizinischen Informationssystemen, S. 93-122. Verlag Vieweg, Braunschweig - Wiesbaden 1995.

[26] A. Krtschil, I. Schmidtmann, J. Schüz, J. Michaelis: Bericht über die Pilotstudie zum Krebsregister Rheinland-Pfalz. Technischer Bericht, Tumorzentrum Rheinland-Pfalz, Mainz 1994.

[27] W.H. Mehnert, M. Smans, C.S. Muir, M. Möhner, D. Schön: Atlas der Krebsinzidenz in der ehemaligen Deutschen Demokratischen Republik. Atlas of Cancer Incidence in the Former German Democratic Republic 1978-1982. IARC Scientific Publications No. 106 / BGA Schrift 4/92. International Agency for Research on Cancer, Lyon; Zentralinstitut für Krebsforschung, Berlin; Institut für Sozialmedizin und Epidemiologie des Bundesgesundheitsamtes, Berlin. MMV Medizin Verlag, München 1992. Oxford University Press 1992.

[28] G. Müller-Ettrich (Hrsg.): Fachliche Modellierung von Informationssystemen. Addison-Wesley, Bonn1993.

[29] C.P. Weagemann: Strategy for Information and Image Management in the 1990s. Optical Disk Institute, Boston, Massachusetts 1992.

Organisation of General Practice: Implications for IM&T in the NHS

Mary Hawking MB, BS

Kingsbury Court Surgery
Church Street, Dunstable, Beds LU5 4RS
Email: maryhawking@tigers.demon.co.uk

Abstract. The increasing use of information technology in the NHS has implications for security and confidentiality, and is the subject of widespread discussion. The nature and organisation of general practice in the NHS has implications for the implementation of any information management system involving information technology in general practice. This paper is an attempt to outline the structure of general practice in the NHS, and to suggest factors which may influence the implementation of the IM&T Strategy and any agreed security policy in General Practice — the level at which most confidential patient information is gathered and stored and may be, eventually, transmitted to others.

1 Organisation and Finance of General Practice in the NHS (England and Wales)

In Britain health care is provided by the National Health Service (NHS) The entire population is registered with a GP (general practitioner — primary care physician[1]); access to secondary care, other than in an emergency, is initiated via general practice, and the individual patient's medical record is maintained by their general practitioner and passed from one GP to the new GP when an individual patient moves and registers with a new doctor. 90% of patient/medical care encounters occur in primary care, and the majority of these are in general practice.

The level of computerisation in General Practice is high. In 1993, the NHS Management Executive commissioned a survey of computerisation in GP practices in England and Wales [1]. This showed that 79% of all practices were computerised, and in practices with over four partners, the level was 97% or more. 98% of computerised practices used their computers for registration, 94% for repeat prescribing, and 90% for clinical records to varying degrees.

[1] Fundholding and commissioning add further complications and are not discussed here

In 1993, three systems (VAMP, Meditel and EMIS) were used in over half the practices surveyed. These systems are mutually incompatible, due to differences in file structure, coding systems and drug databases. Computers have been used increasingly in general practice since the early 1980s, and developments until 1990 were driven by the needs and desires of general practices, with no plans for electronic communications outside the practice — or for the future demands of the NHS Executive.

The relationship of general practice to the rest of the NHS differs from that of other sections.

The organisational structure of the NHS changed on 1st April 1996. Regional Health Authorities (RHAs) were replaced by Regional Outposts of the NHS Executive, and District Health Authorities (DHAs) and Family Health Service Authorities (FHSAs) were combined to form Health Authorities (HAs). This reorganisation was supposed to improve accountability, reduce bureaucracy and complete the reorganisation of the NHS after 1990 into purchasers and providers.

All GPs function as providers and some are also purchasers — GP Fundholders (GPFHs) — for a limited number services. Total fundholding — covering all services, including emergencies and community, is being piloted. Unlike other providers, GPs are, and have been since the beginning of the NHS in 1948, "independent contractors". This means that an individual GP contracts to provide "usual medical services" to patients registered with him/her 24 hours a day and all year. Payment for this is based on the amount awarded by the Doctors and Dentists Review Body.

The majority of GPs work in small partnerships of up to ten or eleven partners; there are significant numbers of single handed practitioners, particularly in inner cities and rural areas, and more than six partners would be considered a large practice. Average list size is around 1900 patients, but this does not allow for the 10% of GPs who are part-time principals.

2 Internal organisation of general practice

General practice differs from all other sectors of the NHS in the methods of recruitment, training, organisation and finance.

GPs are independent contractors, operating single-handedly or in small partnerships from premises owned or rented by themselves, and employing their own staff. Within limits imposed by their Terms of Service and the Statement of Fees and Allowances (the Red Book), they are free to organise their own practices themselves — and this has always been one of the attractions of general practice. This freedom has been restricted by the changes imposed in 1990.

2.1 Recruitment and Training

When a partnership vacancy occurs, the remaining partners decide whether to look for a replacement and obtain approval from the MPC (Medical Practices Committee). It is only in the case of a single handed practice becoming vacant that the HA (Health Authority) has any control over who is appointed: acceptance onto the HA list of a partner selected by a practice is virtually automatic. GPs have to have successfully completed a three year vocational training. Naturally, GPs tend to be appointed for reasons other than IT skills.

A number of factors are influential in the appointment of new partners. These include training, skills, compatibility and personality; computer skills, although welcome, are unlikely to be a major factor, either for selection as a partner or in the compulsory vocational training. If there is any computer experience during either undergraduate or vocational training, it would probably concentrate on the use of available software, rather than issues of technical security. The majority of practising GPs, especially the senior partners, entered general practice before the widespread use of computers. Many GPs neither like nor trust computers — and few believe in the IT (information technology) competence of other organisations in the NHS.

While it is not essential for the partners to be highly skilled in IT, there is a problem in recruiting and retaining IT staff. Each practice has a particular set of software — usually a GP system with or without additional commercial software — so that most training has to be performed at practice level. In addition, a computer manager in general practice has to be familiar with the financial and organisational structure of general practice. The continuing downward pressure on staff budgets ensures that remuneration for IT staff in general practice is considerably less than elsewhere, and likely to remain so. This has implications for the ability of general practices to implement external connections — or, indeed, to make maximum use of existing computer capabilities.

2.2 Confidentiality and data stability

GPs have always been a concerned about confidentiality. If, as seems probable, the responsibility for ensuring confidentiality rests with the person who originally collected the information, there would seem to be little advantage to the average GP in allowing any routine access to the medical records held in the practice, with the ever-present risk of breaches of confidentiality. The incompatibility of existing electronic patient records (EPR) leads to doubts as to whether it is possible to transfer more than simple structured messages — such as registration and item of service (IOS) links with the Health Authorities, and laboratory results — in the foreseeable future.

2.3 Finance and the Review Body

The arrangements for the remuneration of GPs are complex, and poorly understood even within the NHS. As these arrangements are a factor in most management decisions made by GPs, understanding them is important in assessing the impact of IT and security arrangements within general practice.

The Review Body and Intended Net Income: each year, the independent Doctors and Dentists Review Body takes evidence from the GMSC (General Medical Services Committee of the BMA — British Medical Association) and the Department of Health (DOH) regarding the intended income of GPs for the coming year, — the target or intended remuneration — and the level of non-reimbursed expenses needed to run a practice. This last is based on a sample of GP income returns from three years previously.

These two sums are added together, and the "claw back" (the amount by which total earnings of GPs in previous years exceeded the intended remuneration, spread over a number of years by a complicated formula) is deducted. This is then multiplied by the number of GP principals, and divided among the various fees and allowances in such a way that the "average" GP would receive the intended remuneration + expenses – clawback.

This method ensures that, over the years, it is impossible for the total intended remuneration to be exceeded — however much the services performed exceed expectations.

Reimbursable expenses and GMS: some expenses are partially or totally directly reimbursable. These are paid out of GMS (General Medical Services) which covers staff, premises and computers in varying proportions. Computer reimbursement is limited to a maximum of 50% of cost and maintenance for non-fundholders, and 75-100% of fundholding software and hardware for fundholders (some of this is financed from the "management allowance"). As this pool is cashlimited, excessive expenditure on any one element decreases the funds available elsewhere. The maximum staff reimbursement is 70%, and this percentage is falling as levels of reimbursement fall behind the actual increases.

Additional funding for GP/FHSA Links was made available at national and regional levels; the level of linkage in different areas largely reflects the extent to which this was made available to GPs. As far as I know, no additional funding was provided for suppliers' software development costs.

Profits: (i.e. partners' income) is income – expenditure. This means that any increase in expenditure decreases the GPs' take home pay. This does not encourage expenses not deemed to be essential to the running of the business.

2.4 Computerisation in General Practice

General Practice is probably the most highly computerised sector of the NHS — but all these systems were developed and implemented to help the individual practice, and not with the aim of communicating with other parts of the NHS. The result of the early introduction of computers into general practice was that many different systems were developed, using different coding systems, drug databases and filing structures.

At present, up to 40% of data may be lost if a practice decides to change computer systems. Even if changes could be made so that all current systems were able to exchange uncorrupted information, the problem of large amounts of historical data stored in obsolete coding systems would remain. Mapping has proved to be a difficult problem, and it seems that some change in clinical data may be inevitable in mapping [2].

Although the vast majority of general practices are computerised (79% of all practices and over 97% of practices with over 4 partners in the 1993 survey), the extent to which the computer is used in consultation is not known — and anecdotal evidence suggests that it may be much less than assumed by the DOH.

The method of financing computerisation in general practice means that the software development costs to general practice systems of new DOH initiatives are paid, wholly or in part, by the end users out of partnership profits, unless directly financed by the DOH.

2.5 Staff, GPs , computer literacy and IT resources

- Many GPs — especially senior partners — qualified or entered general practice at a time before computers were common. GP systems and coding are not always easy to use, and if the practice has a well organised paper record system, computers may prolong the consultation without any apparent return.
- Some practices have one or more GPs who refuse to use the computer in consultation.
- Most practices use computers for administration and repeat prescriptions — fewer in consultation — and very few have abolished paper records.
- GP computer systems are complex , and are introduced into a working environment where there is unlikely to be any computer system management expertise. The financing of staff in general practice means that it is difficult to recruit staff with IT skills, and to retain those trained on a particular system within the practice. More highly paid jobs with career development prospects are available with the suppliers and elsewhere.
  This means that GPs are dependant on suppliers' support to a far greater extent than most other organisations. The quality and availability of this

support varies between different suppliers and at different times; a common factor appears to be that any major changes, either in software or number of users, leads to a deterioration of support.

2.6 Perceived costs and benefits of IT and especially external linkages

- Financial costs. GPs pay (out of profits) for:
  - at least 50% of computer hardware and maintenance
  - at least 30% of staff time and training costs
  - significant communication costs due to the need for telephone and modem use for supplier support
- Benefits:
  - increased efficiency in claims (this assumes adequate organisation in both practice and HA)
  - ready identification of unregistered patients
  - ability to search for potentially missed financial opportunities
  - ability to produce information demanded by the NHS Executive, e.g. Band 3 data such as numbers of smokers and amounts of alcohol consumed.
- Time. GP and practice nursing time may be increased by:
  - use of the computer in consultation — especially if paper records need to be maintained in parallel
  - need to constantly review organisation and systems within the practice to take maximum advantage of investment in expensive computer systems.
  - increased use of clinical time in IOS and Lab Links
- GP time may be decreased by:
  - computerisation of repeat prescriptions
  - ready availability of previously entered information
  - with IOS Links, fewer signatures
- Ancillary staff time and training may be saved by:
  - potentially less time spent on locating, filing and maintaining MREs (Medical Record Envelopes). This assumes progress towards a totally or partially "paperless practice"
  - quicker and more efficient call/recall systems
  - with GP/FHSA Links, fewer forms to complete
- Ancilliary staff costs include:-
  - additional skills needed for new functions.
  - additional time if letters are to be entered to enable a complete EPR (electronic patient record) to be maintained.

3 Comment on cost/benefit considerations

The degree to which a computer system is seen to be advantageous in an individual practice depends to a large extent on whether previously existing paper based systems satisfied the professional, organisational and financial needs of that particular practice and could continue to do so in the face of increasing demands for information handling. This is, in part, a function of the volume of information needing processing — which in turn depends on the size of the patient population served.

Although many single handed practices are computerised, others find their paper-based systems very satisfactory, and see little advantage in computerisation, whereas virtually all partnerships with more than three partners claim to be computerised. This does not, however, necessarily mean that the computer is used in every or any clinical encounter.

4 Security

Security and confidentiality have always been a factor in General Practice, and it is arguable that implementation of successful policies may be easier within general practice than in larger organisations. There is always a trade-off between total confidentiality and patient safety — but the ready accessibility of information such as repeat prescriptions on screen leads to added practical problems in ensuring that practice policies are enforced: enforcing strict policies may increase risks to such patients as diabetics on insulin and in coma, when timely information may be important to the welfare of the patient.

Having instant access to some information demands stricter protocols and more rigid enforcement of the same.

5 Electronic communication outside the practice

From the point of view of the individual practice, the risks of electronic communication with other NHS and non-NHS organisations, both with regard to confidentiality and data integrity are clear. Apart from a few specific applications, such as GP/FHSA IOS (item of service) and lab links, the benefits are less apparent. The costs, both in time and money, of additional investment in staff, training, equipment, and development and support costs of system suppliers are likely to be considerable.

Until the benefits of linking clinical systems to a wider network become apparent, there is unlikely to be a "business case" for the majority of practices to install outside linkages: non-connection would certainly decrease the risk of breaches in confidentiality — but would also prevent the full development of "person-based information systems" as envisioned in the IM&T Strategy.

To take a homely analogy — to introduce a vehicle transport based system, there are several requirements: vehicles, people trained to operate them, a secure highway and a useful destination.

From the GPs' point of view, we have, to a greater or lesser extent, the first two — and use our vehicles as tractors in the homestead. The highway looks decidedly unsafe, and the usefulness of the destination unproven.

6 Summary

General practices:

- are small organisations — partnerships vary between 1 and over 10 partners
- lack IT expertise
- computerised to serve the internal needs of the practice
- if computerised, mostly use their computers to assist in running the individual practice
- use different systems which are mutually incompatible.

Furthermore:

- the organisational and payment structure mean that an expense has a direct effect on individual partners' incomes
- increased access to patient information increases the risk of breach of confidentiality
- the direct benefits of external electronic links at practice level are unlikely to outweigh the risk and expense

The organisation and funding of general practice leads to a number of potential problems when the issues of electronic communication and transfer of personal medical information are considered. The risks and costs of electronic communication can be identified: the benefits at an individual practice level are less evident.

Abbreviations

BMA British Medical Association
DOH Department of Health
GMS General Medical Services. Used to describe GMS funds — a cash-limited sum covering general practice expenses in premises, staff and computing
GMSC General Medical Services Committee — BMA committee representing general practice
GP/FHSA Links electronic links between GPs and Family Health Services Authorities. FHSAs were amalgamated with DHAs (District Health Authorities) on 1.4.96 to form Health Authorities (HAs)
FHSAs prior to 1.4.96, these bodies managed general practice, dentists, pharmacists etc; DHAs dealt with secondary care
Registration GP/FHSA Links for patient registration
IOS (item of service) Links for transmitting claims for payment of items of service performed to the HA
Lab Links electronic links between practices and laboratories for the transmission of laboratory results
The Red Book the GPs' terms of service and the statement of fees and allowances
IT Information Technology
HA Health Authority (formed on 1.4.96 as noted above)
IM&T Strategy — information management and technology strategy of the NHS Executive, launched in 1992 and relaunched in 1994
MREs Medical Record Envelopes, also known as Lloyd George envelopes. A5 sized envelopes used to maintain patient records in general practice.
NHS National Health Service (England and Wales). There are some organisational differences between the NHS in England and Wales and the NHS in Scotland: this paper refers to England and Wales.
MPC Medical Practices Committee. Controls the number of GPs in any one area according to population needs

References

1. Computerisation in GP practices 1993 survey NHS Management Executive.
2. Mary Hawking, *Code conversions, data stability and the future — an agenda for discussion*, Journal of Informatics in Primary Care June 1995 pp 3–5

Practical Protection of Confidentiality in Acute Health Care

Miss Ruth Roberts, Lecturer; Dr Joyce Thomas, Senior Lecturer in Public Health Medicine; Mr Michael Rigby, Honorary Lecturer and Professor John Williams, Director, School of Postgraduate Studies in Medical and Health Care, University of Wales Swansea

Introduction

The British Medical Association (BMA) document, entitled "Security in Clinical Information Systems"[1], is welcomed for the high profile it is giving to the debate on the many issues involved. However, it is a matter of some concern that the document, although consultative, is widely assumed to be the agreed position of health care professionals.

The document covers security and confidentiality, more than its title suggests, but security and confidentiality are not synonymous, and neither one subsumes the other. "How to Keep a Clinical Confidence"[2] provides a dictionary definition of confidentiality, and the Royal College of Obstetricians and Gynaecologists states that, in the practice of its particular branches of medicine, there are areas deemed especially sensitive. The College, therefore, distinguishes between the definitions of the words "confidentiality" and "security" as follows:

- security concerns the mechanism of keeping any form of medical record free from the risk of unauthorised access or accidental disclosure

- confidentiality is the concept which prevents disclosure of information given in confidence, or of identity, unless the information is necessary for treatment prevention, medical research, or as a statutory requirement[3].

Furthermore, the BMA publication does not appear to have given in-depth thought to the many locations of patients, including the community, which is out of step with the present ethos of the British National Health Service; and it makes no reference to the disadvantages to the care of patients caused by restriction and inefficient sharing of personal health information.

This paper will particularly focus on the acute hospital and the proposed principles. It will attempt to address these with an evidential and scientific approach, as the document takes the luxury (which the BMA would criticise in others) of postulating principles and practice without evidence or analysis.

Organisation of health care within the United Kingdom

Health care in the United Kingdom is supplied, in the majority, by the National Health Service (NHS) and in part by the private sector. The principle of the NHS is that health care should be free at the point of delivery and revenue for the NHS is allocated by Parliament. The United Kingdom consists of four countries, England, Northern Ireland, Scotland and Wales, each country having its own Secretary of State and Health Department.

The 1986 Resource Management initiative[4] in acute hospitals had a principal objective of providing patient based management and clinical information which was accessible by all participants, based on credible data collected from operational systems. It is perhaps not generally realised that each of the four UK countries produced its own Information Management and Information Technology Strategy, setting a framework for the development of information systems, including computerised systems. The Information and Information Technology Strategic Direction for the NHS in Wales[5] and its Technical Strategy and Implementation Programme[6] were published in December 1989 and December 1990 respectively. England launched its Information Management and Technology Strategy, "Getting Better with Information"[7] in December 1992, and Scotland is currently reviewing its strategy. Last year Northern Ireland reviewed its strategy and produced a three year strategic planning framework for the development and use of information and information systems in the health and personal social services[8].

The UK health care professional organisations such as the BMA provide support and advice to its members and need to keep abreast of each country's strategies.

Involvement of the professions

There has been a double vacuum in England with regard to debate of the relevant issues, namely:

- lack of a steering committee or consultation process for the formulation of the NHS Information Technology (IT) Strategy, but with major decisions being made by those who are not in the health care professions

- lack of general debate among professionals, although the Royal College of Physicians has looked at education and informatics, and the Royal College of Psychiatrists undertook a study of mental health information systems, and organised `The Black Hole' Conference in 1994, but there was no follow-up.

There has been some feedback from the clinical professions in relation to the Information Management and Technology Strategy for the NHS in England. The Royal Colleges of the medical profession formed the Colleges' Information Group (CIG) and, in 1995, the nursing professions formed the Nursing Professions Information Group (NPIG), which brings together representatives of the professional organisations, that is, the Royal College of Nursing, Royal College of Midwives, Health Visitors Association, Nursing Specialist Group of the British Computer Society, and two observers from England's NHS Executive Nursing Division and the NHS Information Management Group. NPIG is currently involved in a project to develop training material for nurses focusing on security of computer held patient information[9]. More recently the paramedical professional groups have formed the Clinical Professions Information Advisory Group (CPIAG). In 1991, the Strategic Advisory Group for Nursing Information Systems (SAGNIS) was set up, with the remit of influencing and providing input to England's NHS Information Management Group on the overall development of information management and technology. The Chief Nursing Officer, Department of Health, chairs SAGNIS, and membership includes nurses from the service, representatives from the nursing professional organisations and members of the Information Management Group (IMG)[10]. Of the professions, nursing is unique in its degree of advice and consultation, and the provision of a link health professional between the Nursing Division and the IMG.

However, what is really missing from the IMG strategy, and from the BMA document, is the interprofessional lead. It is extraordinary, and quite inappropriate, that the BMA document, which is looking at clinical and therefore multidisciplinary issues, appears to consider medicine, nursing and the professions allied to medicine (PAM) separately in the field of confidentiality and security. Their concerns with regard to confidentiality are the same and, indeed, patient information collected by nurses and PAMs is often of a more personal and sensitive nature than that required by doctors. Like doctors, nurses have a code of confidentiality which states that they must "...protect all confidential information concerning patients and clients obtained in the course of professional practice and make disclosures only with the consent..."[11]. The viability of the audit trail is also of great importance to nurses in order to comply with the requirements of the United Kingdom Central Council for Nursing, Midwifery and Health Visiting[12]. The Council is a regulatory body and is responsible for the standards of these professions. It requires members to operate within the guidelines and, as with other statutory bodies, members can be struck off for not following their code of conduct.

Involvement of the public

It is laudable for the medical profession to act as watchdog by identifying issues, but not for it to act paternalistically. Evidence is needed on what degree of bureaucracy patients want, and what degree of resource diversion, to match what level of risk avoidance. It is our belief that patients are aware, and actually expect and assume, that information is shared more than it is, for the benefit of their clinical care.

The whole debate on privacy and security should be in the public arena, and not only with the BMA and the medical, health professional, informatics and security communities. Patient Groups need to be included to ensure a spectrum of views.

System specification

With any system, its design should be based on factual analysis of the requirement, matched against cost and risk of adverse effect. This principle is defied by the apparent central decision to develop the former Family Health Services Authority / General Practitioner network, which was a messaging system. This will now develop into the NHS Network, without consultation on user requirements. There is an apparent late (and we believe professionally unsought) addition to the specification, to make it an interactive network, allowing interrogation of systems, with the possibility of accessing records without the system owner's or the clinician's knowledge.

This is quite the wrong way round. An essential prerequisite of any information system design is an understanding of the activities which the system is to serve, and the data required, manipulated and produced by those activities. The specification must be professionally led, and only then should appropriate safeguards be built in to protect the specification.

Threats to confidentiality

The BMA document rightly addresses the security methods for two `trusted systems' interacting, and recognises, as we do, that the greater threats are internal, not external; it therefore relates more to patients' rights than to information technology.

We agree with the BMA's concern about the net effect of information processing, whether the medium is electronic or paper. All the security principles which the document proposes are relevant to manual systems with paper records as well as to electronic records; electronic records should therefore not be singled out adversely, without evidence of their benefits, and without overall risk analysis comparing paper and electronic records.

Disturbing breaches of confidentiality in the United Kingdom and the United States of America are cited in the BMA document. It would be just as easy to find scare stories relating to paper records as to electronic records; not to mention the disadvantages to patients of lack of availability of information. It would be valuable to have such impartial evidence commissioned and included in the debate. It would include analysis of waste of resources and risks to patients of uninformed decisions, delayed treatment and unnecessary duplicate diagnostic tests.

Another threat is the erosion of the patients' privilege for the sake of administrative convenience. We believe that `need to know' must be redefined as a clinical, not administrative, definition, including intention and proof; and that the focus must be on the duty of care that needs to be discharged by the sharing of information.

With regard to the potential threats to confidentiality of electronic records, we would comment that computerised Family Health Service Authority Registers have been running for ten years with the sensitive information referred to in the document, which is now suddenly seen as unethical. It should be noted that the Electronic Patient Record (EPR) Project concerns only hospital records at present, and has nothing to do with General Practice records. The General Practice market in electronic records is in the private sector, and they could be accessed without General Practitioner (GP) or patient consent. The EPR needs appropriate safeguards, but not hints of malpractice.

Practical issues in gaining informed consent to creation of hospital records

In order to give a factual analysis relating to the BMA proposals, we have recent data from a typical local acute hospital trust. The practical difficulties in obtaining informed consent from those patients who are comatose, confused or distressed must be taken into account in any proposals, and not be underestimated. 70% of the trust's admissions were emergencies and only 30% were planned. Of the emergency admissions, 51% were via Accident and Emergency, 40% were from the General Practitioner, 3% were admissions direct from Out Patient clinics, 1% were following a Consultant's domiciliary visit and 4% were via other means.

During 1995/96, 19.5% of total admissions were of the elderly (over 75 years), and 6.2% were aged under 15 years. The over 75s accounted for 31% of the emergency admissions and, of these emergency admissions, 49% were admitted by their General Practitioner and 41% were admitted via Accident and Emergency.

Most patients are anxious about a routine admission to hospital, while an emergency admission is a particularly anxious period for both the patient and relatives. Their main concerns are with what is happening and what is going to happen, and this level of anxiety and concern can act as a barrier or filter to information given during the admission period. One of the authors has been involved with several audits of patient care; one aspect of the audit related to patient safety and included observation of ward activities and specific questions to patients about safety aspects, such as use of the nurse call bell. The majority of the patients spoken to could not remember whether any instructions had been given to them on how to use the call bell system, yet it had been observed that all patients, regardless of whether an emergency admission or routine admission, were instructed immediately on admission to the ward. (Following the audit, ward procedures altered to include repeat instructions the day after admission.) Information on how to contact a nurse is of immediate interest to patients, while access control to their record is likely to be of less interest, therefore even less assimilated.

The BMA document does not discuss the difficult area of confidentiality procedures when the patient is a minor, and sees them as unimportant. We perceive them as very important, and safeguards with regard to children, and also the mentally handicapped and mentally ill, who are not in the acute sector, need to be tackled. We refer to them here, knowing that others will be addressing these issues in detail.

Timing of patient consent to access control list

When a General Practitioner (GP) refers a patient for an outpatient consultation, the letter is used by a clerk to enter patient data onto an administration system. Depending on the needs, the patient's details are recorded against a clinic waiting list or an actual appointment time. A letter is generated, informing the patient of the situation. At present this is undertaken without patient consent, and one must question at what point in this outpatient process, and by whom (hospital doctor or GP), patient consent to the proposed access control list should be obtained.

The practicalities of when to obtain consent also need to be considered by a local Trust which provides an open-access endoscopy service, where the General Practitioner refers patients for the procedure without an outpatient consultation. Prior to admission, the Day Ward Clerk or Officer Manager enters the patient details from the referral letter. Immediately following the procedure (whilst the endoscope is being cleaned), the endoscopist enters the clinical data onto the computerised system, selects the appropriate report and checks and signs the printed letter, which is then posted to the GP the same evening. The endoscopist spends no more than three minutes on this total process, as the patient's demographic and administrative details, plus GP details, are already on the system. The improved communication with GPs about patient care is a major benefit of the system and the service.

Effects on professional duties

The above scenario illustrates that use of this particular clinical information system has not impeded the normal working practice of the endoscopist.

In today's NHS, healthcare professionals' first reaction to the obtaining of consent and setting up the access control list by clinicians is likely to be, "How will this affect my normal working practices?" With 70% of admissions being classified as emergencies, assessments, investigations and the delivery of clinical care are a priority. Although the document refers to "the consultant in charge of a hospital department", in reality these activities, especially the setting up of the access control list, may well be delegated, and nursing is the most likely clinical profession to whom the consultant would wish to delegate the tasks. This will not be viewed favourably, as it will cost nursing time, detract from the delivery of clinical care, and place the nurse in the firing line for adverse patient/relative reaction.

The principles of the security policy proposed in the BMA document

Operational principles can be put forward ethically as practice policy proposals only if they have been subjected to examination as to need, reasonableness and effect, and the

BMA proposed principles fall short of an analysis based approach. Our analysis of these aspects is in relation to the acute hospital view in particular, not least because it is in hospital that effective information handling is most essential for patient care.

Principles 1 and 2

- **Each identifiable clinical record shall be marked with an access control list, naming the people or groups of people who may read it and append data to it. The system shall prevent anyone not on the access control list from accessing the record in any way.**

- **A clinician may open a record with herself and the patient on the access control list. Where a patient has been referred, she may open a record with herself, the patient and the referring clinician(s) on the access control list.**

  Comments

  - Access control lists might work in general practice, but would be hugely difficult to construct accurately for a patient passing through secondary care.

  - These proposals require more detail. The access hierarchy must refer to **items** of information, not just the whole record. There must, therefore, be additional protection within the structure of the medical record, and the cultural issues for the shared record must be tackled.

  - The point of record creation, and validity of consent under conditions of stress or distress, need very careful consideration, as does the financial and staff cost.

Principle 3

- **One of the clinicians on the access control list must be marked as being responsible. Only she may alter the access control list, and she may only add other health care professionals to it.**

  Comments

  - It is difficult to envisage the practical method of allocating and ensuring responsibility, and passing it on.

  - We agree that there are issues to be discussed with regard to computer print-outs conforming to defined standards.

Principle 4

- **The responsible clinician must notify the patient of the names on his record's access control list when it is opened, of all subsequent additions, and whenever responsibility is transferred. His consent must also be obtained, except in emergency or in the case of statutory exemptions.**

Comments

- The costs versus the benefits must be assessed, together with the sociological and ethical issues.
- There is a need to define a clear method of emergency access of records, perhaps allocated to Accident and Emergency (A&E) Departments. This would need a working party of A&E Consultants to define what essential information must be released, eg diabetes and other critical safety information.
- As previously noted, one local trust has 70% emergency admissions, and these patients are not likely to place a high priority on being informed of the names on the record's access control list. Consideration needs to be given to deciding at what stage following an emergency admission informed patient consent should be obtained.
- In clinical audit, outcome requires linkage, and decisions need to be made on obtaining consent at which stages.

Principle 5

- **No-one shall have the ability to delete clinical information until the appropriate time period has expired.**

Comments

- Agreed.

Principle 6

- **All access to clinical records shall be marked on the record with the subject's name, as well as the date and time. An audit trail must also be kept of all deletions.**

Comments

- The need for a complete audit trail is strongly endorsed.

Principle 7

- **Information derived from record A may be appended to record B if, and only if, B's access control list is contained in A's.**

Comments

- An individual has the right to decide what information is to be kept secret, and the law is always on the side of the individual in protecting their right to confidentiality.

- The question of `discrete flags' for sensitive information needs further debate. They can be more injurious or stigmatising than the data they may be perceived to conceal.

- There is a network of obligations regarding information exchange, including those of patients, which have to be negotiated between the patient and the carer.

Principle 8

- **There shall be effective measures to prevent the aggregation of personal health information. In particular, patients must receive special notification if any person whom it is proposed to add to their access control list already has access to personal health information on a large number of people.**

  Comments

  - Clinicians must remember that public health and epidemiology are important in their own right, not only individual issues. Research must not be disassociated from `health' in people's minds.

  - It is unethical to prevent the aggregation of anonymised data for public health purposes of value to all, and safeguards must be found. Decisions need to be made as to the level at which patient identity is screened out, so that the power is not lost to aggregate patient beneficial data. An identifiable record does not mean the same as revealing the identity of the patient.

  - Similarly, it must be recognised that there are instances where named data are essential for epidemiological studies which monitor public health, eg cancer incidence around potentially carcinogenic sites. Without confidence that data are complete, rather than biased by an undefinable non-consenting subset, such studies are impossible; and the same argument applies to cross boundary audit and outcome studies.

Principle 9

- **Computer systems that handle personal health information shall have a sub-system that enforces the above principles in an effective way. Its effectiveness shall be subject to evaluation by independent experts.**

  Comments

  - The need for a sub-system that enforces security is strongly endorsed.

  - The reference to the work of Griew and Currell[13] on the security complexities of patient-based record systems is welcomed.

- We are disappointed that the document does not address how computer systems can themselves be the agents of enforcing and monitoring security. The debate, so far, has implied that access is either total or else denied, and that all data is homogenous as regards sensitivity, concepts which were discarded as unsophisticated in health service computing a long time ago. There needs to be effective research and debate on design and operation of the computer-enhanced security that is needed, with the well-known controls of:
    - differential access
    - data stratification
    - monitoring of abnormal patterns of access
    - presentation of the audit trail as a subset of patient records.

Conclusion

Confidentiality and security are vital issues, and the objectives behind the principles proposed in the document are generally welcomed. Patients have a right to expect the NHS to give them care that is effective and any health care development now must be evidence based; effective measures to ensure confidentiality and security must have the same evidence base as all other interventions. The principles themselves as enunciated for the real world must be considered as not proven, as they do not quantify the adverse effects of their implementation on health and health care, balanced against a quantifiable risk of harm in their absence. Nor does the document provide, or consider, problem analysis and scrutiny of the costs and effects of implementing the proposals, which are key professional principles; nor the means of implementation, which pose great practical difficulties in an organisation as complex as the National Health Service.

The principles should be regarded as the catalyst to further, wide debate, to define a balanced view of the benefits and disbenefits to patients and to consider the effects of alternative solutions. The identification of these solutions is not the exclusive domain of doctors, as much profession-specific personal data are recorded, for example in patient care plans, and all the health care professions must be involved. We also emphasise that research will need to be commissioned in some areas to provide a more empirical analysis of the potential risks and the effects of solutions, in order to inform this debate.

Glossary

A&E	Accident and Emergency
BMA	British Medical Association
CIG	Colleges' Information Group
CPIAG	Clinical Professions Information Advisory Group
EPR	Electronic Patient Record
GP	General Practitioner
FHSA	Family Health Services Authority
IMG	Information Management Group
IT	Information Technology
NHS	National Health Service
NPIG	Nursing Professions Information Group
PAM	Professions Allied to Medicine
SAGNIS	Strategic Advisory Group for Nursing Information Systems
UKCC	United Kingdom Central Council for Nursing, Midwifery and Health Visiting

References

1 Anderson RJ. Security in Clinical Information Systems. British Medical Association, London: 1996.

2 Darley B, Griew A, McLoughlin K, Williams J. How to Keep a Clinical Confidence: A Summary of Law and Guidance on Maintaining the Patient's Privacy. HMSO, London: 1994.

3 Royal College of Obstetricians and Gynaecologists. Statement On Confidentiality; RCOG, London: 1982.

4 Management (Management Budgeting) in Health Authorities. Health Notice, HN(86)34, Department of Health and Security, London: 1986.

5 Welsh Office NHS Directorate. Information and Information Technology Strategic Direction for the NHS in Wales. Welsh Office Publicity Unit, Cardiff: 1989.

6 Welsh Office NHS Directorate. Information and Information Technology for the NHS in Wales: Technical Strategy and Implementation Programme. Welsh Office Publicity Unit, Cardiff: 1990.

7 NHS Management Executive Information Management Group. An Information Management and Technology Strategy for the NHS in England - Getting Better with Information; Department of Health, Leeds: 1993.

8 Management Executive. Strategic Planning Framework for the Development and Use of Information and Information Systems in the Health and Personal Social Services 1995 - 1998 (unpublished).

9 Royal College of Nursing. Information in Nursing Group Newsletter March 1996; Royal College of Nursing, London, 1996.

10 Moores Y. Keynote address; The British Computer Society Nursing Specialist Group Conference, Eastbourne, 1992.

11 United Kingdom Central Council for Nursing, Midwifery and Health Visiting. Exercising Accountability; UKCC, London, 1992.

12 United Kingdom Central Council for Nursing, Midwifery and Health Visiting. Standards for Records and of Record Keeping; UKCC, London, 1993.

13 Griew A, Currell R. A Strategy for Security of the Electronic Patient Record. Institute for Health Informatics, University of Wales Aberystwyth, 1995.

Clinical Systems Security Implementing the BMA Policy and Guidelines

Allan Hassey, Mike Wells*

*Department of Physics, The University of Leeds, Leeds LS2 9JT, England
Tel. +44 (0)113 233 2339, Email. m.wells@leeds.ac.uk

Summary

The Fisher Medical Centre is a highly computerised general practice based in Skipton, North Yorkshire. We decided to try to implement the BMA interim guidelines on maintaining security in computerised patient information systems. This paper outlines the management processes by which a modified set of the BMA guidelines have been implemented in our practice. We also assessed the effects of implementing the nine principles outlined in the BMA security policy document. We describe the problems that we faced, the solutions we found and some of the issues that we were unable to resolve.

Introduction

The Fisher Medical Centre (FMC) is a first-wave fundholding practice of 13,500 patients based in Skipton and Gargrave, North Yorkshire. The practice has been "paper-less" for 18 months and is heavily dependent on its EMIS computer system for patient-records, practice administration, GP-links and laboratory-links. Our computer supplier, the GPs and the practice manager are able to access the system remotely, via dial-up and a modem. The practice is involved in the teaching of medical students and GP training. One partner (AH) is the GP Computer Adviser for North Yorkshire Health Authority.

We have been keenly anticipating the electronic NHS heralded by the development of the NHS-Wide-Network (NWN). However, we did have concerns about the security and confidentiality of patient information, particularly once it had left our practice. The publication of the BMA policy and guidelines helped us to focus our concerns and provide a yardstick against which we could assess our own performance and develop a practice policy.

The FMC has developed, implemented and tested a full recovery of our clinical computer system from system failure or data loss. All our staff have received training in the use and abuse of the clinical information system, the relevant legislation and their ethical and contractual responsibilities.

Set against our security concerns and policies is the need to share patient information. One of the major difficulties in a large practice is communication. There is often a need to share patient information within the practice between GPs, practice nurses, health visitors and district nurses. The primary care team may also include other community staff (e.g. physiotherapists, community psychiatric nurses) as well as other agencies (social services, housing, public health etc.) We have always shared information with other health professionals and agencies when we have believed this to be in our patients' best interests. This disclosure has not always been with the fully informed consent of the patient, but has developed as an ad-hoc arrangement based on mutual professional trust and respect. With the implementation of a "paper-less" clinical information system it has become much easier to share information. We have a primary care team policy of using a single clinical care record which is shared between the different members of the team. We believe this enhances the care that patients receive but accept that this can pose a threat to confidentiality. Our system does not allow restricted access to certain parts of the clinical record. However, we have developed a system of named confidential text files within each clinical record. These are owned by the patient and relevant professional. Nobody else has authorised access.

The publication of the BMA's security policy and guidelines[1,2] stimulated a lively debate within the practice about our own security and confidentiality, the threats we faced and the possible solutions. There was strong initial scepticism about the feasibility of implementing the BMA guidelines. We were aware of NHS Executive guidelines on the protection and use of patient information[3] and emerging international standards[4,5] . We decided to enlist the advice of Professor Mike Wells (MW) as an independent IT expert to help us explore the implications of the policy and guidelines for us.

The FMC is organised so that partners each have several areas of management responsibility. Partners may form small working-groups of two or three with the practice manager for such areas as finance, fund-holding, staff , teaching and training. The computer group is the largest of all with four partners, our practice manager and honorary expert (MW). This group began work to develop our own security policy in January 1996.

> *"The top priority in the guidelines is to return calls when asked for information over the phone or fax. Most actual attacks on patient privacy involve false pretext phone calls."*
> *"The top priority in the policy is to ensure that systems respect the principle that the patient must consent to information sharing."*
> *Ross Anderson - personal communication 22nd Feb 1996*

Training

The practice computer group realised very quickly that further training for doctors and staff was an urgent and on-going priority. We decided to develop a training package that covered the main areas of the guidelines and policy with the help of our IT expert (MW). The training package would be developed by the computer group and implemented by one of the partners (AH) and the practice manager. They would jointly take responsibility for supervising training sessions, disciplinary procedures and practice protocols.

The main areas to be covered in the training program would be:

- What's the problem?
- Confidentiality & security
- Relevant criminal law
- Relevant civil law
- Relevant codes of practice
- Vulnerability and threats
- Safeguards
- Guidelines
- Practice policy

We would approach North Yorkshire HA and our computer supplier to ask for their advice about our training program and offer them the opportunity to contribute to it.

So far we have had one training session for the members of the practice computer group. We plan to extend the training to all our doctors, nurses and staff over the next three months.

It is our belief that there is a parallel need for training throughout the NHS. This particularly involves hospitals where medical staff, nurses, other health professionals, technicians, ancillary and administrative staff all come into contact with confidential patient information. We have asked the Northern & Yorkshire Local User Representative group (LURG) to consider holding a training day for clinicians and NHS managers interested in discussing the issues involved.

BMA clinical system security: interim guidelines

The BMA guidelines provide good interim advice to practices about threats to clinical confidentiality. The main threats are:

- Careless disclosure
- Equipment theft and loss
- Access control
- Communications security
- Disclosure to third parties

The partners decided to try to implement the BMA's interim guidelines in each of these major areas.

Careless disclosure

Our existing practice policy was largely in-line with the suggestions. However, we felt there was room for improvement particularly in our use of fax transmissions. We have adopted all the main suggestions under this heading and details can be found below in the discussion on the BMA policy & principles.

Equipment theft and loss

The practice has an active back-up computer system, consisting of a second main server linked across a network to our main practice network server. The second machine actively backs-up the first in real-time with a delay of 20-30 seconds. The second machine is on a separate floor, at the opposite end of the building in a locked room. Our data is backed-up onto a DAT tape system every day. A number of tapes are kept on and off the premises. We have tested a full system (hardware & software) failure and recovery.

Access control

We use a mixture of terminals, PCs and laptops to provide access to the clinical system. There are no default passwords left in circulation and all doctors, nurses, staff and attached staff have their own unique passwords. There is a quick and simple method for logging in and out of terminals and no excuse for leaving a live terminal unattended.

We have strengthened our access control procedures to ensure that all redundant passwords are deleted and that terminals are *always* left logged-out. We have implemented a system of spot-fines for offenders, with all donations going to a worthy cause. We have removed all default passwords from the system and sought guarantees from our supplier about their security procedures when they log-in and out of our system. The practice is considering the feasibility of an external penetration test to assess our password security.

Communications security

The FMC practice computer system is installed at our two surgery sites, linked by dedicated BT land-line. Our computer supplier, the doctors and the practice manager all have remote access to the system via a modem and dial-up link. Dial-up access is strictly regulated and restricted to the partners and practice manager. Nobody else knows the telephone number or access passwords. No members of staff can get into the building at unauthorised times without the main practice alarm being activated.

We do have a *RACAL Healthnet* connection, which we use for GP-links (registration and items of service) and laboratory results (Lablinks). All incoming files can be screened to check their validity before integration into the computer record system.

We do have Internet access from the main surgery. This is only accessible from a separate PC, unconnected to the practice computer system. It is strictly forbidden to upload any third-party software onto the main practice computer system.

Disclosure to third parties

We do not share or disclose our computer records with any third parties. Social services, Government agencies, the police, solicitors and others *may* be given access to a print-out of relevant medical information with an accompanying report, subject to consent being provided by the patient. We do assume that patients wish us to complete reports for the Benefits Agency and others where it is clearly in the patients' best interests for us to complete the report. We will normally record the report in the medical record and inform the patient at his next consultation. Where we are in doubt, we will try to specifically obtain consent to disclose.

BMA security policy principles

- Access control
- Record opening
- Control
- Consent & notification
- Persistence
- Attribution
- Information flow
- Aggregation control
- Trusted computing base

We decided that the next stage was for us to evaluate our clinical information systems against the BMA's nine principles of data security.

Access control

Current status

Our EMIS computer system cannot implement an access-control list as defined by Anderson. Any user with a valid password can access any part of the system and change or delete any information contained within the clinical records. The EMIS system does keep a full audit-trail of who has changed or deleted records, but it does not keep track of those viewing information. We do not currently maintain paper records for any patients at the FMC.

Proposed changes

We would design a practice leaflet that listed the groups working within the FMC who might reasonably be given access to the patient records. This will be accompanied by a questionnaire to ask patients their views about how we hold and use their confidential medical information.

Every individual member of each access group must have their own unique password. A patient registering with the practice or requesting information will be given this leaflet outlining our access control policy and his right to withhold consent to information sharing. He will also be told that all our clinical records are held on the practice computer system and we will not normally hold separate records on paper or other media. We will also make it clear that there are practical limits to the degree that confidentiality can be implemented by the computer system alone and that we have to rely on our ethical, legal and contractual obligations to enforce it. In exceptional circumstances and with the agreement of the partners, we may consider starting a separate confidential paper-based medical record.

Record Opening

Current status

Our EMIS clinical system does not support different levels of access and hence different access control lists with different groups for different problems. We are entirely dependent on the capabilities of our GP computer system The facility to operate detailed access controlled lists does not exist.

Proposed changes

We have decided to provide patients with information about their computer medical records via the leaflet mentioned above. This will give details of record access and access control.

Control

Current status

The partners assume full responsibility for the care and content of the computer clinical records. Records can be opened by practice staff before the patient has been seen by a GP. A clinical record is started whenever a patient registers. A notification of registration is also passed electronically to the health authority the same day. We already operate a policy of obtaining informed consent for disclosure to third parties. Occasionally we do provide reports without explicit consent (e.g. to the Benefits Agency) where it is clearly in our patients' best interests to do so.

Proposed changes

We will continue to take full responsibility for the computer clinical records. We will reinforce our staff training to emphasise that only GP principals or their nominated deputies (e.g. GP trainees) can assume the responsibility for control. We believe that all partners should share this responsibility equally so that any breach is the responsibility of that individual rather than the registered or usual GP who may not have been involved in any such breach. We believe that this is a more sensible approach for general practice where all the partners are equal Principals in clinical practice. An individual named clinician would seem to suit the hospital / consultant-led model rather better. We will also include information about control on the new confidentiality leaflet.

Consent & notification

Current status

All GPs and everybody who works in the practice and has a valid password has full access to the practice computer system. We cannot restrict authorised access to the system. All our clinical records are on the practice system and we have no alternative method of record storage. We believe that keeping separate medical records is fraught with risks for the patient and that generally a patient's best interests are served by his medical record being available to an authorised member of the practice who may need it.

Proposed changes

We have developed a system for storing a hidden text file in the computer clinical record. This can contain all relevant consultations where a patient has explicitly asked for complete confidentiality. If the patient is still unhappy, then this file can point to a separate paper record. The file will be clearly marked private, with the access control list attached as the document title. Unfortunately, we cannot stop users browsing files, and we have no "view-only" audit-trail. This means that our only means of enforcement is through an agreed code of conduct for all those working in the practice. We are already using this system for patients receiving psycho-sexual counselling. The text file does not form part of the computer medical record and will not be included in any print-outs from the computer clinical record. The text file is not audit-trailed in any way by the practice computer system.

Our staff have been instructed not to answer any enquiries by telephone or fax about patients unless they know they have the patients' consent to do so. (e.g. "Is my wife finished yet so I can pick her up?"). All requests for information about patients will be refused unless we know we have the patients' informed consent and we know who we are talking to. In an emergency, staff are instructed to contact the duty doctor for advice. The doctor will take responsibility for any disclosure and make an entry into the clinical record of that patient. All disclosures made to third parties will be recorded in the clinical records and mentioned to the patient when they next consult or immediately if we are suspicious. We have implemented a call-back policy for disclosure to third parties requesting information, and these numbers are checked against local or national directories. We did not feel it was practical to notify every patient on a regular basis of every disclosure. This is a large administrative burden for the practice and there was no enthusiasm for it amongst the partners.

Persistence

Current status

All entries made in the computer clinical record are kept forever. This is very useful for students and others who regularly attend the practice, but are registered elsewhere. All records are audit-trailed for editing or deleting the record and the trail shows who was logged-in to the system, the date and time of any alteration and the alteration itself.

Proposed changes

We intend to continue with the current system. We believe this works well for us and our patients. (We are aware that this may be a breach of the Data Protection Act's sixth principle). We do not allow deletions from the record unless an entry has been made in the wrong patient's clinical records. Then the deletion must be made by a partner, noted in the record and the patient notified when he next consults. We are also seeking an assurance from our supplier that our system meets the requirements of RFA3.

Attribution

Current status

We do not have a full audit-trail that records "read" accesses. All other entries or edits are audit-trailed.

Proposed changes

Our GP computer supplier is not likely to provide any additional audit-trailing facilities unless they are specified in the RFA. We have encouraged all our staff to log-out whenever they leave a terminal, and we have imposed a system of fines for offenders.

Information Flow

Current status

We do have patients who have expressed concerns about confidentiality and access to their medical, nursing or other records. We assure patients that they can have a confidential relationship with their professional carers but that some entries must be made into the clinical record. These entries can point to a separate paper record if necessary but some reference to its existence *must* be recorded in the main clinical record.

Proposed changes

Our current systems seem to be broadly in-line with this principle and we do not propose any change at this time. We have also developed the facility for a hidden-text file to be included in the computer clinical record and we hope that patients and professionals will use it in preference to separate paper-based records.

Aggregation Control

Current status

We only have access to 13,500 active clinical records on our computer system. We will only provide identifiable aggregated patient data to the health authority in line with registration changes and item-of-service (IOS) claims in accordance with the Statement of Fees and Allowances (SFA). We do take part in audits and research projects from time to time. No identifiable patient data is allowed to leave the practice without the relevant informed patient consents.

Proposed changes

We have spoken to our health authority about submitting anonymous data for IOS claims. They have never received such a claim and do not know whether their software or auditors would accept it. Our computer system will not allow an incomplete form to be submitted to the HA, so we cannot test this any further. Our confidentiality leaflet covers disclosures to third parties.

The trusted computing base

Current status

Our present GP computer system is incapable of implementing the BMA principles in full

Proposed Changes

We have asked our supplier to consider implementing the principles. They are unlikely to do so unless they can make a business case following changes to the RFA and computer reimbursement system. One of the partners (AH) has been invited by the NHS Executive (Information Management Group) to comment on the development of the accreditation processes for GP software. He has already begun discussions with the IMG.

So what have we achieved?

We have tried to implement the BMA guidelines and assess the impact of the security policy in our practice. This process has involved all the doctors, attached and employed nurses and our own staff. We have taken advice from an independent expert (MW) and had discussions with the local health authority, our computer supplier and the NHS Executive (IMG). We have produced a patient information leaflet and a are undertaking a survey to get patients' views on the storage and use of their confidential medical records. We are developing a training package for the surgery and have begun the training process with the practice computing group. This process will continue and will become an integral part of our ongoing staff training and appraisal.

We have begun to recognise the inherent threats and vulnerabilities that exist within the way we work. Where we can make specific changes we have done so (e.g. our hidden computer record and access control list).

There has generally been enthusiastic support from everybody at the FMC for the changes we have made. We regard the guidelines and policy as having acted as a catalyst to long-term change within the practice; this is no "one-off" project.

What have we not done?

There are a number of areas that are outside our control. These lie particularly in the following areas:

- GP-links (exchange of named patient information e.g. Registration & IOS claims)
- Fundholding (patient details accompany clinical details. We do not have confidence that the "safe-havens" standard will adequately protect patient confidentiality).
- Trusted computing base (to implement this will require changes to the various GP computer system accreditation standards - RFA, fundholding & GP-links, as well as a firm link to systems reimbursement to ensure GPs purchase *only* accredited systems).

There may also be more subtle "cultural" factors at work. In our practice, there was little enthusiasm from the partners for us to make changes that could reduce practice income. One partner said to me:

"If patients don't like me sending their contraceptive claim to the FHSA, then perhaps we shouldn't tell them!"

The self-employed status of GPs means that they have to consider the various conflicting calls for investment within the practice. If a new more secure computer system is going to cost a lot of money, then who pays? This is particularly difficult where there is no consistent system of computer systems reimbursement linked to standards. Another GP asked me:

"If it came down to a new more secure computer system or your skiing holiday, which would you choose?"

The consensus was that the practice computer system was important, but not *that* important.

We believe that the NHS Executive, the BMA and the computer systems suppliers must tackle these areas together. Individual practices, health authorities and GP system suppliers cannot be expected to craft any meaningful policy by themselves. We look to our national representatives to provide the necessary leadership and all those involved to co-operate in that process.

References

1. Security in clinical information systems: BMA Publications 1996. ISBN 0 7279 1048 5
2. Anderson R. Clinical systems security: interim guidelines. BMJ 1996;312;109-111.
3. The Protection and Use of Patient Information: Dept. of Health. 1996.
4. Smith MF. Data protection, health care, and the new European directive. BMJ 1996;312;197-8.
5. Standards Australia (1995). Standard: Personal privacy protection in healthcare information systems.
6. Hawker A. Confidentiality of personal information: a patient survey. Journal of Informatics in Primary Care 1995; March:16-19.

Appendices

Patient Confidentiality Leaflet

FISHER MEDICAL CENTRE

Privacy & Confidentiality of Your Medical Records.

1. Your medical record is a life-long history of your consultations, illnesses, investigations, prescriptions and other treatments. The doctor-patient relationship sits at the heart of good general practice and is based on mutual trust and confidence. The story of that relationship over the years is your medical record. At The Fisher Medical Centre, we store *all* our patients' medical records on our practice computer system.

2. Your GP is responsible for the accuracy and safe-keeping of your medical records. You can help us to keep it accurate by informing us of any change in your name, address etc. and by ensuring that we have full details of your important medical history. We take regular action to protect your records from accidental loss or damage. We keep secure "back-up" copies of all our computer records.

If you move to another area or change GP, we will send your medical records to the health authority to be passed on to your new practice. However, we will keep a copy of all entries into your records whilst you were registered with us.

A) YOUR RIGHT TO PRIVACY

You have a right to keep your personal health information confidential between you and your doctor. This applies to everyone over the age of 16 years and in certain cases to those under 16. The law does impose a few exceptions to this rule, but apart from those (listed in detail below), you have a right to know who has access to your medical record.

B) WHO ELSE SEES MY RECORDS?

There is a balance between your privacy and safety, and we will normally share some information with others involved in your health care, unless you ask us not to. This could include doctors, nurses, therapists and technicians involved in the treatment or investigation of your medical problems.

This practice is involved in the teaching of medical students and the training in General Practice of young doctors. If you see a medical student or GP trainee during a consultation, they may be given supervised access to your computer medical record.

Our practice & district nurses, midwives and health-visitors all have access to the medical records of their patients. It is our policy to have a single medical and nursing record for each patient. We firmly believe that this offers the best opportunity for delivering the highest quality of care from a modern primary care team.

Our practice staff have limited administrative access to the medical records system. They notify the health authority of registration and claim details and perform various filing tasks on the medical records.

All our doctors, nurses and staff have a legal, ethical and contractual duty to protect your privacy and confidentiality.

C) WHERE ELSE DO WE SEND PATIENT INFORMATION?

We are required by law to notify the Government of certain diseases (e.g. meningitis) for public health reasons.

The law & Coroners' courts can also insist that GPs disclose medical records to them. Doctors cannot refuse to co-operate with the courts without risking serious punishment. We are often asked for medical reports from solicitors. These will *always* be accompanied by the patient's signed consent for us to disclose information. We will not normally release any details about other people that are contained in your records (e.g. wife, children, parents etc.) unless we also have their consent.

Limited information is shared with health authorities to help them organise national programmes for public health such as childhood immunisations, cervical smear tests and breast screening.

GPs must keep the health authorities up to date with all registration changes, additions and deletions. We also notify the health authority of certain procedures that we carry-out on patients (contraceptive & maternity services, minor operations, night visits booster vaccinations) and other "item-of-service" procedures, where we are paid for performing these procedures.

Social Services, the Benefits Agency and other Government agencies may require medical reports on you from time to time. These may not include your signed consent to disclose information. Failure to co-operate with these agencies can lead to patients' loss of benefit or other support. We will normally assume that you wish us to complete these reports in your best interests unless you specifically ask us not to do so.

Life Assurance companies frequently ask for medical reports on prospective clients from the GP. These are *always* accompanied by your signed consent form. GPs must disclose *all relevant medical conditions* in the report unless you ask us not to do so. In that case, we would have to inform the insurance company that you had instructed us *not to make a full disclosure* to them.

D) HOW CAN I FIND OUT WHAT'S IN MY MEDICAL RECORDS?

We are required by law to allow you access to your computer and written medical records. If you wish to see your records, please contact our practice manager, Mrs Jenny Hutchinson, for further advice. All requests to view medical records *must* be made in writing to the surgery. We are allowed to charge a small fee to cover our administration and costs.

You can contact Mrs Hutchinson by calling the surgery on Skipton 799622.

We have a duty to keep your medical records accurate and up-to-date. Please feel free to correct any errors of fact that may have crept into your medical records over the years. After all the records are *yours* and it is important that they are as accurate as possible!

E) WHAT WE WILL NOT DO!

To protect your privacy and confidentiality, we will not normally disclose any medical information over the telephone or fax unless we are sure we are talking to you. This means that we will not disclose information to family, friends or colleagues about any medical matters at all, unless we know that we have your consent to do so.

This also means that we will not normally disclose test results over the phone and may wish to call you back to ensure that we are talking to the right person.

Our staff will not disclose any details *at all* about patients over the telephone. Please do not ask them to - they are instructed to protect your privacy above all else!

Finally, if you have any further queries, comments or complaints about privacy and your medical records, then please contact Jenny Hutchinson at the surgery or talk to your own GP.

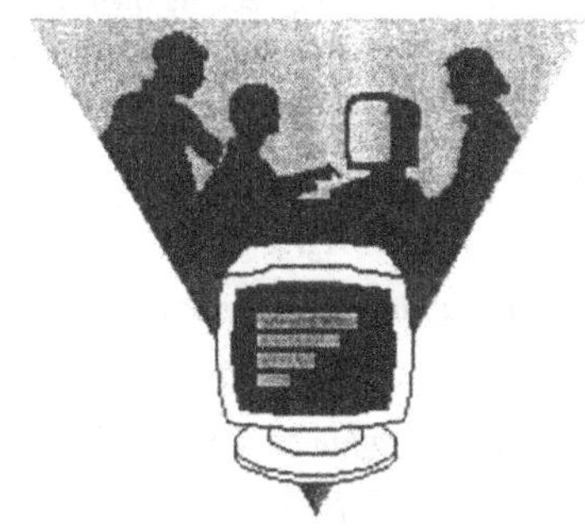

Patient Questionnaire

This survey is being carried out jointly by the Practice and Professor Mike Wells of the University of Leeds. We want to discover your attitude, as a patient, to some important aspects of the introduction of computerised Medical Records. Please answer the following questions. Tick the box to show whether you agree or disagree with the statement at the start of each question.

Questions 1 and 2 are about whether or not you should be able to insist that the Practice does not keep your medical records on a computer, and on the possible effects this might have on you. Keeping your records on a computer means that they will be more readily available to those who are treating you, but may mean that they can be more easily accessed by other people.

1 I should give my consent before my medical records are kept on a computer system

Agree ☐ Neutral ☐ Disagree ☐

2 It is more important that my records should be readily accessible than to protect my privacy

Agree ☐ Neutral ☐ Disagree ☐

Questions 3 to 6 are about the extent to which Doctors, other Medical staff, and the non-Medical staff of the Practice can read and alter your medical records. Restricting access to your medical records will help to ensure that they remain private. However, on occasions it may cause difficulty in treating you, or in routine administration.

3 My medical records should be kept private between me and the doctors in the Practice

Agree ☐ Neutral ☐ Disagree ☐

4 Nurses and other medical staff in the Practice should be able to read and alter my medical records

Agree ☐ Neutral ☐ Disagree ☐

5 Non-medical staff in the Practice should be able to read my medical records

Agree ☐ Neutral ☐ Disagree ☐

6 Non-medical staff in the Practice should be able to alter my medical records

Agree ☐ Neutral ☐ Disagree ☐

Questions 7 to 9 are about the extent to which staff of NHS Hospitals can read and alter your medical records kept in the Practice. When your Doctor refers you to a Hospital he sends only the information that he regards as necessary to allow the staff of the Hospital to treat you. The Hospital will, of course, keep its own records about your treatment by the Hospital. There may be occasions on which the staff of the Hospital could treat you more easily if they had access to your medical records.

7 Medical Staff in NHS Hospitals should be able to read my medical records in the Practice

Agree ☐ Neutral ☐ Disagree ☐

8 Medical Staff in NHS Hospitals should be able to alter my medical records in the Practice

Agree ☐ Neutral ☐ Disagree ☐

9 Non-medical Staff in NHS Hospitals should be able to read my medical records in the Practice

Agree ☐ Neutral ☐ Disagree ☐

Questions 10 and 11 are about the extent to which administrative staff of the NHS can read and alter your medical records. Administrators may need to know details about you, for instance in dealing with screening for cancer, or in order to produce statistics about health risks.

10 Administrative staff in the NHS should be able to read my medical records

Agree ☐ Neutral ☐ Disagree ☐

11 Administrative staff in the NHS should be able to alter my medical records

Agree ☐ Neutral ☐ Disagree ☐

Questions 12 and 13 are about the extent to which the NHS may pass details of your medical records to others. There may be occasions in which it would be helpful to pass your medical records from the NHS to other parts of Government, for instance in dealing with sick pay or disability pensions. There may be occasions in which it be helpful to pass your medical records to non-Government organisations such as drug manufacturers or insurance companies.

12 The NHS should be allowed to pass my medical records to other Government agencies

Agree ☐ Neutral ☐ Disagree ☐

13 The NHS should be allowed to pass my medical records to non-Government organisations

Agree ☐ Neutral ☐ Disagree ☐

Personal Details

Some details about you. Please tick the box for the answer to each question. If you do not wish to answer these questions, please ignore them

P1 What is your age in years?

Under 15 ☐ 16 to 25 ☐ 26 to 45 ☐ 46 to 65 ☐ Over 65 ☐

P2 What sex are you?

Male ☐ Female ☐

P3 Are you here as a Patient, as the Parent or Guardian of a child, or as a Carer for an elderly or incapacitated person?

Patient ☐ Parent/Guardian ☐ Carer ☐

Comments

Do you have any other comments you wish to make? Please use the space below.

Patient Questionnaire results

Method

The questionnaire was handed to 330 patients attending the Fisher Medical Centre over a two-week period during May 1996. The questionnaire was accompanied by an explanatory leaflet (Appendix 1). The aim of this study was to give patients information about the security and confidentiality of their medical records and at the same time some idea of the views and concerns of our patients.

We were aware that other research in this area[6] has shown that some patients have concerns about sharing their medical information even within a practice between GPs. These concerns become increasingly common as information is shared further outside the practice and is particularly strongly held where information may be shared with NHS administrators. It is against this background that we undertook our own survey.

Results

147 questionnaires were returned to the practice, representing a response rate of 44.5%. The detailed responses for each question are shown on the form below by percentage response.

The majority of respondents were women (76%) and the age-response rate was fairly evenly spread.

Most patients (57%) felt that they should give explicit approval for their records to be kept on computer, though 61% felt that having their records accessible was more important than protecting privacy (19%).

The results from questions 3 - 6 suggest that patients feel strongly that their records should be kept confidential between them and the GPs, though over half (53%) felt that nurses and other medical staff should also have read/write access to their records. Our patients felt that practice administrative staff should not have read or write access to their medical records (65%).

The results from questions 7 - 9 suggest a very similar set of views about hospital staff access to the GP-held record. Most patients seemed comfortable with hospital doctors having read access to their GP records, but seem evenly divided about whether hospital doctors should be able to amend the GP records. Patients strongly disapprove of hospital administrative staff having any access to the GP record (82%).

Questions 10 - 14 are about sharing patient information with the wider NHS and other agencies. Only 1/3 of our patients felt that NHS administrative staff should have read-access to their records, even for NHS call and recall programs. Patients seem to strongly disapprove of information sharing with other agencies both within (62%) and without (83%) government.

Conclusion

These results are broadly in agreement with other studies and our expectations. Our patients want the following:

- Records to be held on computer only with the patient's consent
- Records to be confidential between the patient and doctor
- Records accessible only to other doctors or nurses within the practice
- Records can be made available to hospital doctors
- Records not to be shared with other agencies

These results will be incorporated into our evolving response to the BMA guidelines and principles.

Patient Survey on Computerised Medical Records

This survey is being carried out jointly by the Practice and Professor Mike Wells of the University of Leeds. We want to discover your attitude, as a patient, to some important aspects of the introduction of computerised Medical Records. Please answer the following questions. Tick the box to show whether you agree or disagree with the statement at the start of each question.

Questions 1 and 2 are about whether or not you should be able to insist that the Practice does not keep your medical records on a computer, and on the possible effects this might have on you. Keeping your records on a computer means that they will be more readily available to those who are treating you, but may mean that they can be more easily accessed by other people.

1 I should give my consent before my medical records are kept on a computer system

Agree 57 Neutral 29 Disagree 14

2 It is more important that my records should be readily accessible than to protect my privacy

Agree 61 Neutral 19 Disagree 19

Questions 3 to 6 are about the extent to which Doctors, other Medical staff, and the non-Medical staff of the Practice can read and alter your medical records. Restricting access to your medical records will help to ensure that they remain private. However, on occasions it may cause difficulty in treating you, or in routine administration.

3 My medical records should be kept private between me and the doctors in the Practice

Agree 74 Neutral 18 Disagree 8

4 Nurses and other medical staff in the Practice should be able to read and alter my medical records

Agree 53 Neutral 21 Disagree 26

5 Non-medical staff in the Practice should be able to read my medical records

Agree 12 Neutral 23 Disagree 65

6 Non-medical staff in the Practice should be able to alter my medical records

Agree 8 Neutral 8 Disagree 84

Questions 7 to 9 are about the extent to which staff of NHS Hospitals can read and alter your medical records kept in the Practice. When your Doctor refers you to a Hospital he sends only the information that he regards as necessary to allow the staff of the Hospital to treat you. The Hospital will, of course, keep its own records about your treatment by the Hospital. There may be occasions on which the staff of the Hospital could treat you more easily if they had access to your medical records.

7 Medical Staff in NHS Hospitals should be able to read my medical records in the Practice

Agree 79 Neutral 9 Disagree 12

8 Medical Staff in NHS Hospitals should be able to alter my medical records in the Practice

Agree 43 Neutral 19 Disagree 38

9 Non-medical Staff in NHS Hospitals should be able to read my medical records in the Practice

Agree 6 Neutral 18 Disagree 82

Questions 10 and 11 are about the extent to which administrative staff of the NHS can read and alter your medical records. Administrators may need to know details about you, for instance in dealing with screening for cancer, or in order to produce statistics about health risks.

10 Administrative staff in the NHS should be able to read my medical records

Agree 33 Neutral 22 Disagree 45

11 Administrative staff in the NHS should be able to alter my medical records

Agree 6 Neutral 18 Disagree 76

Questions 12 and 13 are about the extent to which the NHS may pass details of your medical records to others. There may be occasions in which it would be helpful to pass your medical records from the NHS to other parts of Government, for instance in dealing with sick pay or disability pensions. There may be occasions in which it be helpful to pass your medical records to non-Government organisations such as drug manufacturers or insurance companies.

12 The NHS should be allowed to pass my medical records to other Government agencies

Agree 22 Neutral 17 Disagree 62

13 The NHS should be allowed to pass my medical records to non-Government organisations

Agree 5 Neutral 12 Disagree 83

Personal Details

Some details about you. Please tick the box for the answer to each question. If you do not wish to answer these questions, please ignore them

P1 What is your age in years?

Under 15 2 16 to 25 11 26 to 45 31 46 to 65 32 Over 65 24

P2 What sex are you?

Male 24 Female 76

P3 Are you here as a Patient, as the Parent or Guardian of a child, or as a Carer for an elderly or incapacitated person?

Patient 91 Parent/Guardian 8 Carer 1

User-Oriented Control of Personal Information Security in Communication Systems

Ulrich Kohl

University of Freiburg

Institute for Computer Science and Social Studies

Telematics Department

Friedrichstrasse 50

79098 Freiburg, Germany

kohl@iig.uni-freiburg.de

The security of personal information often competes with the purpose for which the information was acquired and stored. While the intention is to use the data to fufil a certain aim, or to perform an order, security and safety control restrict access to the data in order to exclude access which is not considered to be necessary by all means. Generalized, universal rules often cannot be used to make decisions about the security of personal information. In many cases, individual users of a system are responsible for the security of the data and only they know what has to be done, and what has to be prevented. The approach which gives *them* the ability to decide on security features is called user-oriented security.

This paper describes the requirements that lead to an user-oriented security approach and the requirements that user-oriented security imposes on information and communication technology. Section I illustrates the need for multilateral security and what is lacking in today's security systems to fulfil these needs. Section II examines existing communication systems and security measures and identifies their weaknesses in comparison with face-to-face communication. Then, in section III, a referential collection method for identifying end user security requirements is presented and exemplified by a clinical environment in section IV. Section V concludes the paper.

I Multilateral security as a condition of acceptable technical communication

The upcoming information age implies the involvement of information technology (IT) in nearly every area of human activity. This development is enabled by falling prices, increasing performance and decreasing size of information techology devices and leads to ubiquitous computing, i.e. computers which disappear from peoples' awareness or personal devices which always accompany their owner. In combination with the trend to connect computers to a global network, the impact on economy and society is immense and is currently being discussed using catchphrases such as information highway, global information infrastructure, or information society. The huge amount of information cannot be mastered without the support of information technology.

This development has not only positive, but also negative consequences. As more and more information owned by users and concerning usees is stored on IT systems and becomes potentially globally accessible, this information is also potentially globally abusable. Thus, the aspects of information and system security which have already been under examination for many years now are gaining more and more importance for the security interest groups manufacturers, owners, (network or service) providers, users, and usees.

Today's security measures, e.g. cryptographic algorithms or security protocols, have reached a very high technical standard and systems which are secure in principle can be designed. Nevertheless, the overall security of today's IT systems does not comply to all security requirements of the different interest groups.

In particular, today's security systems tend to protect the requirements of the manufacturers, owners, and providers of IT systems rather than the users' and usees' requirements. The security view is centralized and mainly protects the IT system and its assets against users and third parties, which bears the following disadvantages:

- the systems are secure in principle, but not in practice, because the protection mechanisms are not used properly or not used at all [Mull89],
- the system-oriented security view restricts the functionality of the IT system and handicaps the users' work [PeKo95],
- the security view is unilateral because requirements of important interest groups are neglected [RDLM95],
- and the complexity of all security requirements cannot be administered centrally and in advance.

Security has to take into account the requirements of all interest groups and be multilateral. A multilateral security system supports all requirements and is the prerequisite for the acceptance and use of an IT system by all interest groups. To obtain multilaterality, today's unilateral approach of centralized security has to be complemented with an approach for decentralized, user-oriented security. User orientation yields a decentralized management of the security complex. The idea is that users can specify their own security requirements at any time thereby creating a high degree of flexibility so that the security system can match all requirements in detail.

The combination of system and user oriented security faces several difficulties. The dilemma of competing requirements, e.g. secure billing of a service provider vs. anonymity of a user, has to be resolved by finding a sustainable compromise for all parties. Such a compromise can only be implemented in a designable system. Ideally, no technical restrictions should influence the solution, rather the technology should be able to implement all possibilities, enabling the final implementation to depend exclusively on „political" decisions. On the technical side, static security architectures have to be extended in a way that they are able to handle dynamic specifications during system run-time.

To achieve a multilateral security system, a current system must be extended with a user-oriented part. Necessary steps comprise the analysis of the scope of possible user requirements, a requirement specification scheme as a model for both the user interface and the technical realization, and finally a concept for the dynamic realization of security requirements.

II Security measures in open communication systems

Many problems in computer science are solved by using layered abstraction models, views, or architectures. In the area of communication systems, both proprietary systems like IBM's SNA and open systems like TCP/IP and the ISO Open System Interconnection (OSI) reference model [ISO84] use hierarchical architectures where each layer provides a specific service and offers it to its next upper layer. The definition of an abstract service of a layer allows for constructing different implementations of one layer which can be mutually exchanged. So each real communication system can be configured matching the actual needs, e.g. an OSI system for a single enterprise could consist of twisted pair copper wire network, the token ring protocol for layers 1 and 2, connection oriented network layer, transport layer class 0, basic activity subset session and presentation layers, and an application layer for remote database access. Each layer realization could be replaced by another one without the need to change the rest of the system; e.g. for a change to a coaxial wire layers 1 and 2 had to be replaced by the

CSMA/CD protocols. So different layers can be combined in a manner that they match the requirements posed on the communication system best as possible.

It is clear that is is not feasible to change the combination of layers and their features very often. So only requiremens which can be expressed pior to building the system can be respected. Dynamic requirements which show up during run-time cannot be fulfilled. Furthermore, not every interest group will have a right to influence a system's configuration; the main groups are the manufacturers, owners, and providers of systems. The concept of Intelligent Networks (IN) [CCITT93] makes an effort to respect dynamic requirements on networks. The main idea is to decompose the service of a layer and to define service independent building blocks (SIB) which can be used to combine high-level services in a more dynamic way. The combination is done by specifying a service logic which expresses the order of the initiation of SIBs and the data flow between them. INs have been designed to achieve a greater flexibility for designing new services in public communication systems, e.g. in the area of comfort telephony. Although the configuration of INs and their services is more flexible than in classical layered architectures, users and usees do not have a chance to influence the services directly and interactively.

In the area of security measures many mechanisms have been developed to serve certain purposes. Using a layered view, the lowest layer consists of security mechanisms which issue specific operations on the security relevant objects. Examples of security mechanisms are cryptographic algorithms like DES or RSA, but also authentication protocols, access control procedures and the associated data structures like access control lists. The mechanisms can be seen as basic security building blocks. They are not suitable for being used by users. For users, the security mechanisms have to be combined to provide security services which supply services appropriate for them. This procedure can be interpreted as using a security toolbox like shown in figure 1 [Mart92].

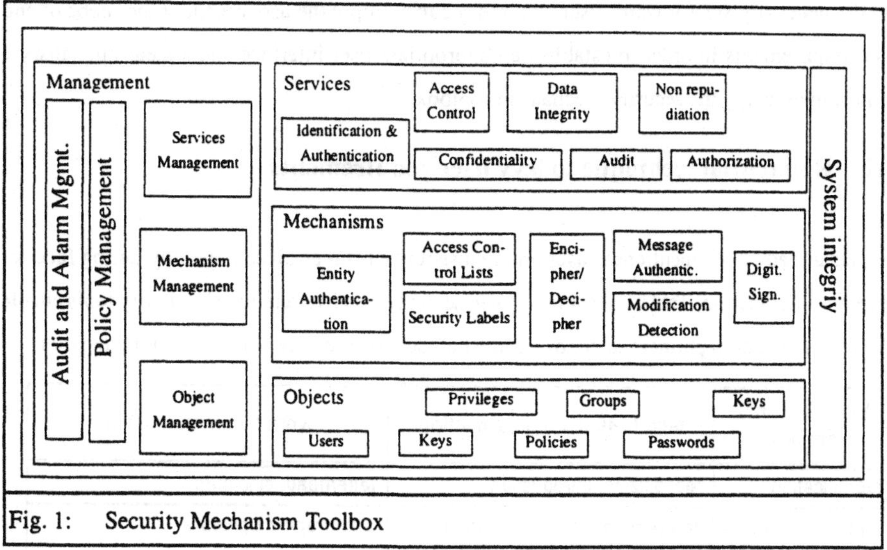

Fig. 1: Security Mechanism Toolbox

The security toolbox concept resembles the IN concept. New security services or service features can be created by defining how a service on user level has to be implemented on the mechanism level. Unlike the IN concept, the procedure of choosing the adequate mechanisms to provide for a desired service which has been described by [BlPf95] does not use a service logic but only hierarchical and static interdependencies.

A system built according to the security toolbox approach is able to provide almost every desired security service. Although, if the IN concept is strictly followed, its disadvantages remain, e.g. that the services have to be designed and implemented in advance and that spontaneous security requirements of end users during run-time cannot be fulfilled, which is a main feature of real user orientation.

A paragon of real user orientation is provided by examining human face-to-face communication. Communicating persons can control all security features of their (e.g. verbal) communication implicitly. To transfer this paragon to technical communication, a separate channel between the communication device and the person has to be established in order to communicate the security requirements. The user interface therefore has to be extended to „understand" the user's requirements. If a requirement is specified, the system has to fulfil it immediately and dynamically which can only be done by means of a flexible architecture.

So the necessary steps towards user oriented security imply the assessment of the scope of end user requirements in order to establish an appropriate user interface and a means to satisfy a requirement using the security mechanism toolbox.

III Referential technique to levy user requirements

As has already been mentioned, user oriented security is takes place implicitly during face-to-face communication. Table 1 shows the basic security services and which security tools enable the communication partners to control almost all security features of their communication.

basic security service	face-to-face communication	written communication
identification	recognizing, introduction	letterhead, signature
authentication	recognizing (voice, appearance)	autographic signature
access control	choice of communication location	physical measures
authorization	implicitly by choosing the communication content	bound to ownership of physical medium
confidentiality	whispering	address remark „personally", secret code, seal, safe
integrity	guaranteed	seal
availability	physical presence	duplication, safe
non-repudiation	testimony of others	justification of autographic signature, registered mail
provability	testimony of others	receipt, opinion of script
anonymity	confessional	anonymous letter
pseudonymity	masquerade	ciphered advertisement
unobserveability	choice of communication location	warranteed using paper mail
unchainability	choice of communication locations	warranteed using paper mail

Table 1: Security tools of non-technical communication

The security features of face-to-face communication are an initial reference for building a catalogue of requirements for technical communication. The scope of the features can be analyzed by constructing scenarios of the working environment where only face-to-face communication is used to communicate and access information.

Genesis of technology often uses a metaphor which can be seen as a model of understanding of the reality that serves as orientation for a system engineer [DHM92]. An example of application of a metaphor is the desktop metaphor, where the real desk and the way work is done at a desk serve as a model for the screen design and the user interface. Modern operating systems use icons to represent the different objects like files (texts), directories (folders), programs (e.g. a pen representing a word processor), or logical devices (printer or waste bin). A user works with the icons by carrying out actions, such as double-clicking, or drag-and-drop, which emulate operations in the real world like picking up a pen, or putting a paper in a folder.

When the metaphor is derived directly from the real world, it is possible that the technical solution will not be optimal because restrictions existing in the real world are emulated, although an alternative technical solution could overcome the restrictions. For example, digital signatures are superior to written signatures in some respects. Under the premise that real world restrictions can be abolished by means of a technical solution, facts and processes of the real world can be reinvented, so the resulting ideal of the real world which at the outset ignores certain restrictions which do not appear in the technical equivalent is better than a metaphor for obtaining requirements for the technical solution.

In the case of communication systems, technical communication is superior to face-to-face-communication in two dimensions: time and place. Whilst face-to-face communication requires all communicating persons to be at the same place at the same time, technical communication is able to bridge distance and to establish an asynchronous communication channel. On an abstract level of view, technical communication enables persons to communicate with other persons and access information anywhere and anytime.

Therefore, the ideal of the reality, which serves as a reference for investigating the users' security requirements, has to ignore the restrictions of face-to-face communication – just modelling their implicit security control features – and has to model an environment where face-to-face communication and access to information are possible from every place at all times. This implies an environment in which all possible persons and the information store are located in a restricted area and present all of the time. In such an environment, every wish to communicate can be executed immediately by talking to the communication partner. Written information is located in a central store and, as a result, omnipresent. Access to this data can be granted under permanent supervision of the responsible person. Scenarios in this ideal environment serve as a reference for requirements a technical communication system has to satisfy.

IV Scenarios in the ideal hospital

Following the ideal , a hospital is reduced locally to a single floor where all the staff and the patients reside as a work group permanently, as illustrated in Fig. 2. Rooms serve as offices for physicians, locations of special services such as the radiology department, and as hospital rooms for the patients. The patient document store is located centrally, so every access request can be served immediately. As unlimited access is not intended, the store can be modelled as a cabinet with lockers where each locker contains one patient's data. Each patient has a treating physician who is responsible for the data and holds the key for the specific locker. Each access to his patient's data requires that the treating physician is asked to come to the locker and unlock it.

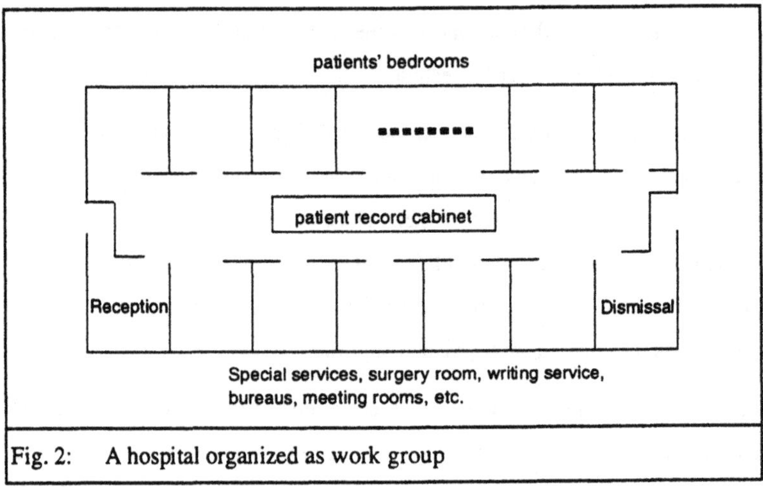

Fig. 2: A hospital organized as work group

As every communication process is face-to-face, all basic security services are present according to Table 1. Identification and authentication are achieved by assuming all persons in the hospital know and recognize each other. Access control and authorization are realized through the responsible physician's permanent control of the locker and the data and his physical presence during each access. Confidentiality is reached by locking the data. Integrity and availability are implicitly provided by the medium and the type of storage. Non-repudiation and provability areachieved by protocolling and confirming every access.

The detailed end user security requirements result from the analysis of scenarios of typical hospital processes in the ideal environment. They can directly be transferred to a real hospital environment and a real hospital information system because the need for information exchange and the security requirements are principally independent from organization structure details; they only depend on the medical need. The following scenarios exemplify the modelling of a hospital process within the ideal environment and which security requirements result from the analysis. As a third point it is shown how the user-oriented security features can be realized in a real hospital environment using information and communication technology. It is assumed that all patient information is stored digitally and can be accessed via the network, e.g. by applyong an open document archive like ISO/OSI DFR (document filing and retrieval) [ISO91a, ISO91b].

Reception of a new patient

- Process

  The reception of a patient is the first step of his stay. A record for the patient is created and the historical data of a patient, i.e. demographical and billing data, are added. The patient is assigned to a ward. The last step in the reception process is the performance of the anamnesis, where the medical history of the patient is acquired and added to the record.

- Modelling and security features

  In the ideal hospital, the patient enters the hospital at the reception room. After the creation of the record the staff takes the patient to his room and transfers him and the record personally to his treating physician who finishes the reception process by entering the anamnesis and locking the record in the cabinet.

  Empty records are stored in the reception room where only the reception staff has access; so only they can create new records (3)[1]. The record is given personally (1, 2) from the reception staff to the treating physician who also assumes the responsibility (3, 4, 5). The physical transfer of a paper based medium ensures the integrity (6).

- Requirements on IT support for a real environment

  The creation of a record can be executed electronically by the reception staff. Both creation and entry of historical data are bound to this role. After that, all rights to the record are transferred to the treating physician who can be identified using an electronic directory. With the transfer, all rights of the reception to access the patient's records expire, except the information regarding the room number (if the patient has agreed).

1. The basic security services which are implicit to the described actions are abbreviated (1) identification, (2) authentication, (3) authorization, (4) access control. (5) confidentiality, (6) integrity, (7) non-repudiation, and (8) provability.

Assignment of a consultant

- Process

  A consultant is a physician who is not treating the patient, but who is consulted by the treating physician due to his special expertise. Thus, he has to get the access rights ro read the relevant information from the patient record and to write his counsel.

- Modelling and security features

  A consultant is also located on the ward. The treating physician takes the patient record and visits the consultant. There, they can discuss the problem and exchange the necessary information. If the physical presence of the patient is necessary, he can also come to the consultant's office, or they can visit his room. The consultant writes his counsel and gives it to the treating physician who adds it to the record.

  The communication between the two physicians takes place in the consultant's office, where the treating physician formulates his request and chooses the information he wants to show to the consultant (1, 2, 3, 4, 5). When he leaves, he takes the record back (4, 5). When the counsel is written, the consultant signs it (7, 8) and gives it to the treating physician who adds it to the record (1, 2, 4, 5).

- Requirements to IT support for a real environment

  The treating physician has to formulate his request in a form or via email, which he signs digitally. He transfers the necessary access rights to the patient record to the consultant. The consultant receives the order and the rights, creates his counsel, signs it digitally and adds it to the patient record. After that, all rights expire.

Change of a patient's ward

- Process

  In case of complicated diseases it is possible that a patient has to be readmitted to another ward. In this case, the patient and the patient record are delivered from the old to the new ward. The old treating physician informs the new one about the case and transfers the responsibility and the rights.

- Modelling and security features

  The change of a ward is simple to model. All stations are located on the same floor of the ideal, so the patient himself needs not to be relocated physically. The patient record also may stay in its locker. Old and new physician meet each other (1, 2) and discuss the situation. Responsibility is transferred by giving the locker key to the new physician (3, 5). Posessing the key, the new physician then has all access rights as well as further rights.

- Requirements to IT support for a real environment

  Of course, IT cannot avoid the physical relocation of a patient in a real hospital. The relocation is however supported by the reservation of a bed in the new ward and the coordination of certain circumstances. The transfer of access rights to the patient record has to be issued by the old treating physician who has all rights, including the right to give away his rights. This procedure can be coupled to the transfer of the role *treating physician*.

The scenarios show that in typical hospital processes a high demand on user-oriented security is found. In many cases, only certain persons, e.g. the treating physicians, know what has to be done with the patient and his record. They have to reach decisions dynamically, depending on immediate medical situations. User-oriented securityemerges in all basic security services. Identification and authentication are guaranteed by visual recognition of the communication partners. Authorization is granted spontaneously by showing the record or parts of it to the grantee. The presence of the treating physician implies access control and data integrity, because all actions are supervised by the responsible person. Confidentiality is provided by locking the records in the cabinet. Availability results from the permanent presence of the responsible person and the records.. Non-repudiation and provability are reached through protocolling and autographic signature, respectively. Decisions about the use of security services are not possible in advance and cannot be centrally administered. On the other hand, the ideal environment obviously cannot be directly transformed ino a real environment.

Technical communication can emulate some features of face-to-face communication and, therefore, can be used to port the implicit security features of the ideal to a real environment. An analysis of the security features in the ideal serves a a guideline for the construction of the IT system. Table 2 summarizes the security features of the ideal and requirements for their transfer to technical communication systems.

basic security service	features in the ideal of omnipresent information	Requirements to the transfer on IT in a real environment
identification	personal recognition; done at each communication act	all accesses and operations just through identified actors

Table 2: Security features of the ideal of omnipresent information and their transfer

basic security service	features in the ideal of omnipresent information	Requirements to the transfer on IT in a real environment
authentication	coupled to identification	secure, trustworthy authentication entity for peer authentication
authorisation	direct authorization through reponsible person	flexible delegation of rights through reponsible person
access control	access in presence of responsible person	control of accesses through control of access rights
confidentiality	storage in locked cabinet, delegation just by responsible person	no access without access right; management of access rights through responsible person
(data) integrity	storage in locked cabinet; communication via false-proof media	confidential and manipulation-proof storage and communication of data
confidentiality	autographic signature	digital signature
provability	protocol of accesses by responsible person	automatic protocollation of access wishes and issued accesses according to responsible person's wishes

Table 2: Security features of the ideal of omnipresent information and their transfer

V Summary and outlook

Although communication systems can extend the functionality of direct human communication, today's systems lack the implicit control of security of the processed and communicated information. Security mechanisms can be integrated in the system architecture to overcome this disadvantage. For the integration and the use of the security measures, the end user has to be able to specify his requirements and the system has to be able to comply to the requirements immediately.

This paper presents an approach to ascertaining the scope of user requirements by analyzing the circumstances in an ideal environment. Application of a referential acquirement technique resulted in a catalogue of user-oriented security requirements which need to be fulfilled by technical communication systems.

Applying the security mechanism toolbox metaphor, the IT system architecture can be designed to be flexible, in order to react directly to the users' requirements. A prototype for an information and communication system following the user-oriented approach was built into the SaferCom-project [JKP94], where an open document archive for storing and exchanging patient records based on international standards such as ISO/OSI DFR [ISO91a, ISO91b], X.500 [CCITT92], ECMA TR/46 [ECMA88] and ECMA-138 [ECMA89] was developed [Jure96].

References

[BlPf95] Uwe Blöcher and Axel Pfau: Auswahlstrategien für Sicherheitsmechanismen zur Erfüllung von Sicherheitsanforderungen. Datenschutz und Datensicherheit 5/95, p. 284-292. vieweg 1995.

[CCITT92] Comité Consultatif International Télégraphique et Télephonique: X series Recommendations. X.500: Data Communication Networks, The Directory. Geneva 1992.

[CCITT93] Comité Consultatif International Télégraphique et Télephonique: I/Q series Recommendations I.312 / Q.1201. Principles of Intelligent Network Architecture. Genf 1992.

[DHM92] Meinolf Dierkes, Ute Hoffmann and Lutz Marz: Leitbild und Technik. Zur Entstehung und Steuerung technischer Innovationen. Edition Sigma, 1992.

[ECMA88] ECMA TR/46: Security in Open Systems, A Security Framework. European Computer Manufacturers Association, Geneva 1988.

[ECMA89] ECMA-138: Security in Open Systems, Data Elements and Service Definitions. European Computer Manufacturers Association, Geneva 1989.

[ISO84] ISO/IEC International Standard 7498: Information Processing Systems – Open Systems Interconnection – Basic Reference Model. International Organization for Standardization, 1984.

[ISO91a] ISO/IEC International Standard 10166-1: Document Filing and Retrieval (DFR), Part 1: Abstract Service Definition and Procedures. ISO/IEC, 1991.

[ISO91b] ISO/IEC International Standard 10166-2: Document Filing and Retrieval (DFR), Part 2: Protocol Specification. ISO/IEC, 1991.

[JKP94] Marjan Jurecic, Ulrich Kohl and Ernst Pelikan: SaferCom – ein Prototyp für Datenschutz in verteilten Klinikanwendungen. In: Datenschutz und Datensicherung 3/94, S. 146-152, vieweg 1994.

[Jure96] Marjan Jurecic: Datenschutz und Datensicherheit in offenen Rechnernetzen – eine technische Lösung ausgeführt für den Krankenhausbereich. Shaker 1996.

[Mart92] Raymond J. Martin: IBM Security Architecture: A Model for Securing Information Systems. IBM Corporation, 1992.

[Mull89] Sape Mullender: Protection. In: Distributed Systems. p. 117-132. ACM Press, 1989.

[PeKo95] Günter Pernul and Lothar Kochne: Semantische Objektmodellierung anwendungsorientierter Informationssysteme vom Standpunkt des Sicherheitsmanagements. In: Wolfgang König (Ed.): Wirtschaftsinformatik '95, p. 169-176. physica 1995.

[RDLM95] Kai Rannenberg, Herbert Damker, Werner Langenheder, Günter Müller: Mehrseitige Sicherheit als integrale Eigenschaft von Kommunikationstechnik. In: H. Kubicek, G. Müller, K.-H. Neumann, E. Raubold, A. Roßnagel (Ed.): Jahrbuch Telekommunikation und Gesellschaft, p. 254-261, 1995. R.v. Decker's Verlag, 1995.

Information Management as Risk Management

Beverly Woodward

We are in the midst of a growing international debate over the handling of medical information. The debate is not primarily over technical issues. It is not about whether there exist technical means for restricting access to computerized medical records. Nor is it principally about how best to improve the technical tools for restricting access. The debate is largely a policy debate. It is a debate about the extent to which access to patient records *should* be restricted.

On the one side, there are those who argue that patients have a right to obtain confidential medical care and that health care services should be organized to provide this, even if it is in some ways inconvenient and increases costs. On the other, there are those who argue that tight control over access to personal medical information will impede the provision of good medical care, interfere with research, and hamper attempts to reduce health care expenditures.

Those who favor liberal access policies take two tacks. Either they argue that the goods achieved by relatively easy access to personal information are of greater value than the informational seclusion that will be lost thereby [1] or they argue that privacy should be redefined in such a way that the apparent conflict between the right to confidential medical care and certain economic and professional goals can easily be overcome. When privacy is redefined as "the right to step out in public" or when it is urged that we adopt a model of "privacy as participation" — definitions quite at odds with standard dictionary definitions — the tension between the pursuit of privacy and certain other objectives tends to melt away.

Those who regard privacy and confidentiality in medical care as critically important reject these arguments. They understand the right to confidentiality in traditional terms, as expressed, for example, in the booklet *'Good Medical Practice'* issued by the General Medical Council in Britain. It states: "Patients have the right to expect that you will not pass on any personal information which you learn in the course of your professional duties, unless they agree." The proposed redefinitions of this right are perceived as abrogations of it.

Utilitarian arguments that invoke the social goods that may be attained by liberal disclosure policies are especially unconvincing to those who have experienced serious violations of the right to confidentiality. For the victim of a serious breach of confidentiality there is no common yardstick by which the injury experienced can be compared with the hypothetical social benefits that may be achieved if traditional standards of confidentiality are abandoned.

The Right to Confidentiality

Medical ethicists have long spoken of medical privacy and confidentiality as individual rights. When ethicists employ the language of rights, it is usually with the intention of indicating that a fundamental ethical norm is at issue and that respect for the human person requires adherence to this norm, even though it may sometimes be inconvenient and may interfere with other apparently legitimate goals.

In both medicine and law there are a number of fundamental norms that are considered of paramount importance for professional practice. In the domain of law enforcement, for example, a key norm is respect for the potential innocence of a suspect. Accordingly, the suspect has a right not to be tortured and a right to legal counsel. In the medical domain, a fundamental norm is respect for the autonomy or potential autonomy of the patient. Thus, if the patient is competent, patient consent to treatment must be obtained. Moreover, the patient has the right to seek the advice of more than one professional and the right to make the final decision about which advice to accept or reject. A competent patient may, for example, walk out of a hospital against medical advice, since the hospital is not meant to be a prison.

The right to confidentiality is closely linked to the requirement for patient consent to treatment. Because becoming a patient exposes the individual to harm, touching a patient without consent constitutes battery under the law. While the physical ministrations of medical caregivers render the patient physically vulnerable, the verbal interchange with care providers often creates psychological vulnerability and vulnerability in a wide array of personal, social, and economic relationships. The promise of confidentiality is a means of protecting the patient against the exploitation of the latter sorts of vulnerability and of providing the conditions under which consent to treatment is a rational choice. Respect for the consent requirement therefore implies respect for the confidentiality requirement.

Just as there is always a danger that law enforcement will override its fundamental norms and make the individual suspect a victim of its desire for criminal convictions, so there is always a danger that medical practice will make the individual patient a victim of its desire to manage and direct human behavior or of its desire to advance one or another kind of research. In recent years medical technology, information technology, and business management tools have placed the patient in an increasingly vulnerable position in these regards.

The management and monitoring of patient behavior have often been rationalized (if not justified) as necessary for the patient's own good or in order to prevent the spread of disease, but of late a new factor is frequently invoked–the need to contain medical costs. If current trends in this regard continue, we may be headed for a time in which medical cost containment will be linked to highly intrusive forms of personal surveillance. This can be illustrated by examining a new approach to risk management and its potential impact on patient care and the handling of patient records.

The Master Patient Index

In May 1996 a workshop on the Master Patient Index was held in Santa Fe, New Mexico under the auspices of a number of public and private groups, including the Los Alamos National Laboratory, the Health Care and Financing Administration of the U.S. Dept. of Health and Human Services, the Computer-based Patient record Institute, and Healthcare Open Systems Trials.

The Master Patient Index is conceived as a computer tool that tracks patients across all their encounters with the medical system. In the announcement for the workshop the following statement appeared: "It has been noted that information management is no longer a records management issue but a risk management issue." This provocative statement summarizes several assumptions about the emerging role of personal information in the health care industry in the United States.

The risk management referred to here is management of the financial risks run by medical insurers and providers–basically the risks of losing money or not generating as much income as is considered desirable. The primary goal of medical information management in this context is business management. While the actual goal of private sector business management in the health care industry is often the enrichment of corporations and individuals, the goal that is generally stressed is control of health care costs. This more respectable goal is common to both the private and the public sectors in the United States, although the approach to achieving it is somewhat different in each case.

The Private Sector

The United States has no universal health insurance program. Health insurance is a benefit provided by some, but not all employers. (It can also be purchased by the individual, generally at a rather high cost.) Managed care is the tool of choice of employers for lowering their health insurance costs. It is also the tool of choice of health insurers for increasing their profits. The financial goal of managed care is to influence physician behavior in such a way as to bring about a reduction in the medical services provided. (In the jargon of the managed care industry any funds that must actually be expended on care constitute the 'medical loss ratio.') The method typically used by insurance companies to manage the behavior of physicians and other health care providers has been to threaten not to pay or to refuse to pay for services that they consider unnecessary.

But this cost control method has not been entirely successful, as physicians and hospitals have found ways to resist some of these pressures. More recently insurance companies have hit upon the idea of passing on some of their financial risks to health care providers by using a capitation payment scheme rather than a fee-for-service scheme. Under capitation, physicians and other health care providers acquire a personal financial incentive to decrease the level of services provided and their cost. Because the physician receives a fixed amount per month per "covered life", the financial goal of the physician in such a set-up is to get a large pool of patients who require relatively few services. The fewer the services that are required, the smaller the physician's costs. The larger the pool of patients, the higher the physician's income [3].

Managed care organizations (MCOs) manage the complex relationships between physicians, hospitals and other medical care providers under capitation schemes. Information is considered the key to effective management. The key source of the information that is considered relevant is the patient record. Experts on capitation contracts are now advocating the use of a single record for both administrative and clinical purposes, on the grounds that merged financial and clinical information is required for cost benefit analysis and the management of resources [4]. Such a merged record is, of course, incompatible with a segmented record scheme that controls access on a segment by segment basis.

When records management becomes risk management, information systems are designed to track patients in order to see what each patient is costing. If one reads business newsletters on capitated care (not to be confused with the public relations newsletters that patients receive), one finds statements such as the following: "For providers delivering care under contracted arrangements... patients must be closely tracked across multiple entities to ensure adherence to contracts and to support resource utilization management techniques" [5]. To insure error-free tracking and to prevent fraud, some companies have begun to use biometric identifiers, e.g., fingerprints, to establish the identity of each individual who seeks care.

Biometric identifiers make it possible to avoid name identifiers and may enhance privacy in certain limited respects, since they make it possible for patients to consult medical personnel without using their true names. However, they make it impossible to obtain truly anonymous health care, since the patient is uniquely identified and tracked in the system's records. They also convey to the patient a message of distrust. The patient, if not practicing outright fraud, may be wasting resources.

The control of risk thus leads to patient surveillance. Patient behavior is to be monitored in order to manage costs. Furthermore it is not just the individual's behavior when illness strikes that is to be monitored. Some health care management experts envisage going considerably further. The following quotation is illustrative. "The focus of the MPI [Master Patient Index] within an IDS [Integrated Delivery System] will shift away from a patient focus toward a broader, member or person focus. To reflect this shift, it may be appropriate to modify the terminology so that the master patient index becomes the master person index. This broader definition more accurately reflects the growing needs of health systems in which tracking wellness is a part of the comprehensive care process" [6].

In this vision, managed care becomes comprehensive care, which includes tracking the behavior of the individual even when he or she is not ill and has manifested no desire to interact with the medical system. The rationale for continuous tracking of the person, not just intermittent tracking of the patient (i.e., tracking of illness episodes), may be expressed in terms of benevolent concern.

"XYZ Healthcare is dedicated to your well-being." In internal publications of the managed care industry, however, it is more often expressed in terms of bottom line economics. The individual who is not tracked may one day become an unexpected source of large costs. Any and all facets of an individual's life may be relevant to risk and the management of risk.

The more extensive information obtained by means of continuous monitoring of the person for the sake of the person's "wellness" is unlikely to find its final resting place in the databanks of the health care industry. As noted, in the U.S. there are close links between employers and insurers. The NPI in its various forms is likely to expand employer access to personal information about employees.

In fact employers are already using medical and lifestyle information to attempt to influence and manage the off-the-job activities and behavior of employees. In the words of a recent *Time* magazine headline, "Big Brother Wants You Healthy" [7]. Employee wellness programs are a means frequently used. These programs are often designed not only to encourage health promoting behaviors, but to penalize unhealthy behaviors. For example, employees at one U.S. company must, if they are pregnant, attend childbirth classes, or else lose their insurance. Another company fires any employee caught smoking, whether on the job or at home. The *Time* article says that some experts believe that such programs have already gone too far.

The Public Sector

Lest anyone conclude that all these developments are merely an aberration of the corporate control of medical care and therefore of little relevance when medical care is publically financed, it must be noted that governmental insurance programs and public agencies in the U.S. are also engaged in medical surveillance and have plans for more extensive activities of this kind. The rationale offered is the same–the need to control costs. This tends to be expressed as concern for the taxpayer, always a popular theme.

Both federal and state agencies are currently engaged in medical data collection. Seventeen states are collecting nonaggregated outpatient care data. Six of them — Florida, Maine, Missouri, Pennsylvania, South Carolina and Tennessee — collect the data with Social Security Numbers attached. A number of these states are carrying out or plan to carry out longitudinal analyses of individual patient records, tracking patients over time through episodes of illness and the aftermath of illness. The Health Care Financing Administration, the federal agency which administers Medicare, is assisting such efforts by sharing extensive patient-identified data on Medicare patients with state agencies.

Public health agencies are also designing strategies for gathering comprehensive health-related information. Tn a recent paper linking public health concerns and the national information infrastructure [8], several nationally prominent figures in the public health field advocate the development of a logically integrated health information system in which information collected once will be used for multiple purposes. They assert that "the interests of public health and the health care sector are beginning to converge" and that in the future "health care organizations and the public health community will need to coordinate not only their roles and responsibilities, but their information systems".

The authors advocate the collection of data about the health status, personal risk behaviors, and medical treatment of individuals along with more traditional types of data concerning sources of injury and disease in the environment. The linkage of these kinds of data makes possible correlations of clinical risks with behavioral and environmental factors. Legislation introduced in Congress last year (the Bennett-Leahy bill, S. 1360) would facilitate this development by authorizing the collection of patient-identified data by public health agencies without patient consent.

The collection of extensive personal information puts new forms of power into governmental hands. Not surprisingly these activities and planned activities have generated controversy. In some states the citizenry is relatively unaware of state data collection practices. In others, such as Naryland and Vermont, there has been widespread publicity and opposition. There are concerns about the sale, whether legal or illegal, of the data collected, the purloining of data, and the merging of data bases so as to generate comprehensive profiles of individuals. Antidiscrimination advocates fear that the data may be used to develop governmental policies that are detrimental to one group or another.

New Ethical Challenges

Corporate and governmental medical cost cutters often act in similar ways and have a similar appetite for personal medical information, but the potential impact on the patient and on society differs somewhat. Corporations wield economic power and can manipulate the opportunities of individuals as employees and consumers, while governments can use the power of law, regulation, and ultimately repressive force to coerce and constrain individual behavior in all aspects of life. Government monitoring programs raise the spectre that the time-honored distinction between private matters and public matters will be lost and that ultimately no aspect of life will be free of governmental intrusion.

Virtually no one would argue with the proposition that modern technology has led to runaway medical costs and that this process is not at its end. The rationing of medical services is an issue that has yet to be confronted adequately by ethicists and by the public. In the absence of this discussion, the health care industry and politicians are promoting a technological fix, namely the creation of widespread computerized medical information networks as a means of achieving greater control over the health care system.

Those who advocate the adoption of this technology claim that it is neutral with respect to privacy, or even that it can better protect privacy than paper record-keeping systems. But these claims are misleading. The unique capability of computers is to collect and analyze large quantities of data and to transfer data quickly. That is precisely why their adoption and use in medicine is being advocated. The availability of computers has already generated a host of new data gathering schemes. Privacy measures are resisted because they impede the full-scale exploitation of this far from neutral tool.

Those who are financing the computerization of medical records are not doing so to enhance privacy, even if they pay lip service to privacy concerns. They are doing so in order to exercise greater control over medical expenditures and the medical care process in general. How patients will benefit, if at all, is uncertain. Whether health care cost reductions, if they are achieved, will be passed on to consumers as lower insurance premiums or lower taxes is just as problematic.

Reid Cushman has argued that the widespread adoption of modern information technology in medicine makes the patient a subject in a large-scale experiment [9]. If this proposition is correct, the imposition of this technology, unless accompanied by stringent access controls and access policies, dispenses with two sorts of consent: consent to be a subject in an experiment and consent to a diminution of the traditional right to confidentiality (a right that is linked, as was shown earlier, to the requirement that consent to treatment be obtained). This situation can be remedied only if patients are given the opportunity to decline to have their personal medical information entered into any computerized information system, i.e. , to opt out of the experiment.

Notes

1. See, for example, Lawrence 0. Gostin, "Health Information Privacy", *Cornell Law Review*, Vol. 80, No. 3, March 1995.
2. Paul M. Schwartz, "Privacy and Participation: Personal Information and Public Sector Regulation in the United States", *80 Iowa Law Review*, 1 995.
3. David W. Lee, Ph.D., *'Capitation: The Physician's Guide'*, American Medical Association, 1995.
4. Karen A. Duncan, Ph.D., *'Patient Indexing Strategies for the New Continuum of Care'*, *ComNets*, February/March, 1996, p 27.
5. Randy Golub and John Quinn, "Goals & Roles: Integrated Delivery Systems & the Master Patient Index", *Healthcare Informatics*, November 1994, p 68.6.
6. Ibid., p. 68.
7. *Time*, May 6 1996, p. 62.
8. Roz D. Lasker, M.D., Betsy L. Humphreys, M.L.S., and William R. Braithwaite, M.D., Ph.D., "Making a Powerful Connection: The Health of the Public and the National Information Infrastructure", Report of the U.S. Public Health Service Public Health Data Policy Coordinating Committee, July 6, 1995.
9. Reid Cushman, *this volume*

Responsibility Modelling: A New Approach to the Re-Alignment and Re-Engineering of Health-Care Organisations

Dr. Andrew Blyth

Department of Computer Studies, The University of Glamorgan.
Pontypridd, Mid Glamorgan. CF37 1DL, UK.

Tel. No: 01443 482245, Fax. No: 01443 482715
E-Mail: ajcblyth@glamorgan.ac.uk

Abstract

Health care providers today perceive the adoption and utilization of information technology as vital to their success in the market place. The adoption and utilisation of information technology will change an organisation and will force it to re-align and re-engineer its processes. Within health-care organisations the process of adopting information technology, and re-engineering the organisation, is one that must not fail, as to fail in such a process is to expose people to the risk of death, or at least loss of personal information. It is vital then that when re-engineering in the medical sector we ensure that confidentiality, security and safety polices are not compromised. Recent medical information system failures have shown us that the process of adoption and utilization is far from easy. This has sparked a research debate into why systems development and re-engineering activities are failing. It is therefore vital that we develop techniques that allow us a) to explore and define how an information system is going to change the organisation's structure and behaviour b) to manage the process of re-aligning the organisation's structure with its processes, and c) to demonstrate that the re-aligned and re-engineered structures are still in line with safety and security policies.

1.0 Introduction

Within organisations, large tasks tend to be devolved to groups of people who work together in complex ways to achieve an overall objective [6]. This has always been the case, and yet technical systems design tends to assume a single user with a discrete task. The failure to recognise that users work in a collaborative or co-operative way, and to design systems to support this way of working, can account for the relatively low success rates of many complex technical systems [1]. The design of systems to meet user needs involves the alignment, or re-alignment, of an I.T system with not only the needs of the users, but also the policies and objectives of the organisation. Introducing any system be it technology or human based will change the way the organisation functions. Consequently when developing systems for any organisation the developer must be aware that they are re-engineering the organisation. This re-engineering will necessitate the re-alignment of the organisational processes. Consequently we must validate at the end of the re-engineering activity that the organisation's policies are still valid and adhered to.

The management of any information technology system is something that is driven by a) organisational, governmental and legal policies, and b) the needs, wants and desires of its users [9, 10]. The analysis of recent system failures [3, 4, 7, 8], and information systems in general, [15] has pointed to faults in the gathering of information concerned with the social and organisational aspects of the system as being a major contributing factor to the success or failure of the system. In a recent report [15] only 20 percent of organisations engaging in re-engineering activities are said to show any positive results. In [12] after a survey of information technology in hospitals, the point is made that information must be made more appropriate, timely, accurate and usable. In addition, the information contained in a medical information system is subject to laws and organisational policies concerned with privacy and confidentiality of medical records [11]. Users need access to information - however as pointed out in [13,14] the result of illegal accessing of information can result in fatalities. Thus we need to identify when, where, by whom and under what conditions access to information is required and what policies govern the accessing and manipulation of information. An information system can only be cost effective if it meets all the needs of the system owners and system users and helps them fulfill their policies. The question that we are now forced to ask is "*How do we do that ?*"

One of the aims of my approach is therefore to enable design teams to address these organisational requirements (in particular the alignment of requirements to organisational policies and goals), and thereby to produce IT systems that match not only the organisational and functional needs of the individual end user, but also those of groups of users and their associated usability and acceptability requirements. The requirements identified in order to achieve the aim of supporting different members of the design team are as follows:

- to identify organisational mechanisms or processes for fulfilling critical non-functional requirements.
- to identify the full range of relevant a) user needs, and b) organisational goals and objectives, in a specific organisational context;
- to derive for an IT system appropriate specifications which take account of organisational as well as individual requirements;
- to compare the organisational requirements match of different design alternatives;
- to ensure that the organisational policies such as those concerned with confidentiality, safety and privacy are adhered to.

The method used to determine requirements and align them to the organisation must allow the system designer to explore possible solutions (involving both the IT system and possible organisational change) and their consequences at the same time as specifying the problem, thereby refining the understanding of the problem and developing the solution by an iterative process.

2.0 The Basic Concepts

2.1 The Concept of Agency

My aim is to describe and reason about organisations that embody both a social and a technical system. These however comprise one single system, a socio-technical system, and, as such, cannot be described or modelled in terms of state and behaviour only as a purely technical system might be, since there is a fundamental difference between social and technical systems. It is to be able to differentiate between social and technical objects (i.e. between people and computers) that we introduce the idea of agency. A machine may perform the same tasks as a person, but the person will hold responsibilities for those tasks in contrast to the machine which cannot hold responsibility. The person is said to be an agent and hold the agency.

It is important to realise that an agent is distinct from both an individual human and a role. An agent holds the particular set of responsibilities that comprise an agency. Thus depending on how responsibilities in a social system are allocated and combined, so agencies are composed and decomposed. An agent also differs from an individual in that an individual may hold more than one agency simultaneously. An agent differs from a role in that a role is not merely an agency or a collection of agencies but also includes a set of relationships with other agents. These are structural or social in nature, arising from responsibilities that relate to the other agents.

This concept of agency is one of the strengths to reorganisation of a socio-technical system, since it facilitates the reallocation of agency in a way that takes into account as fully as possible the structural and organisational implications of the change. Since agency is considered as a coherent set of responsibilities, it permits the discussion of issues related to the change in and reallocation of responsibilities when some functions or agents in the system are proposed to be automated.

2.2 The Concept of Role

The concept of role provides us with a powerful and expressive tool [2]. We choose to describe an organisation as a set of related work roles for the following reasons:

- A role is a descriptive concept that can be used to represent many different organisational realities from the formal and structured to the fluid and unstructured.
- A role defines task responsibilities along with what resources are required, and thereby functionality requirements.
- A role defines the relationships between role holders and the behaviour they expect of one another which in turn defines many non-functional requirements.

Hence our concept of role allows us to distinguish: a) an agent with associated obligations such as accountabilities and responsibilities to other agents; and b) activities that interact through information flows and are structured into tasks and operations. This enables us to represent and analyse the relations between these concepts and to represent the way in which they operate in real organisations.

3.0 Modelling Responsibilities

3.1 What is a Responsibility ?

Evidence has shown that the responsibilities concerned with a particular problem, and the agents that hold them, can be a great source of domain knowledge [3,4]. From Figure 1 we can view a responsibility as a relationship between two agents, or stakeholders, regarding a specific state of affairs, such that the holder of the responsibility is responsible to the giver of the responsibility, the responsibility principal.

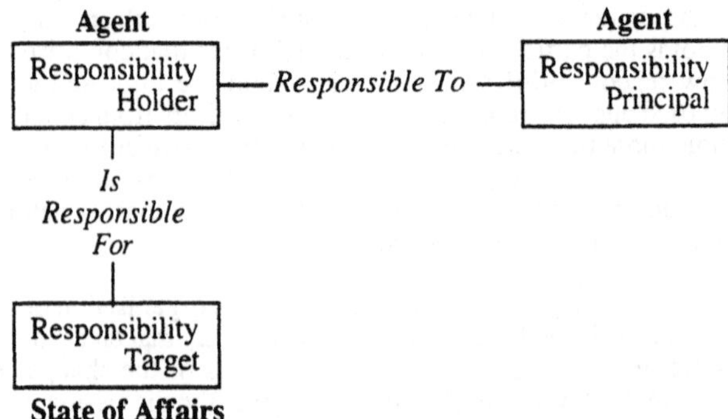

Figure 1 - The Responsibility Relationship

The full definition of a responsibility consists of the following:

- who is responsible to whom;
- the state of affairs for which the responsibility is held;
- a list of roles held by the responsibility holder (how the responsibility can be fulfilled);
- the type of responsibility (these include accountability, culpability, legal liability).

3.2 Responsibilities, Roles and Actions

This brings us to the distinction between responsibilities, roles and actions. We use these concepts in the sense that agents execute actions in order to perform roles imposed on them by virtue of the responsibilities they hold. These roles are what the agents have to do and effectively describe their *'jobs'*. Roles are performed with regard to other agents. Roles are the link between responsibilities that agents hold and the actions that agents execute. Another way of describing this relationship is to say that responsibilities tell us *why* agents do something, roles tell us *what* they do and actions are *how* they do it. The distinction between responsibilities and roles is apparent from the words we use: a responsibility is *for* a state of affairs, whereas a role is *to do* something that will change or maintain that state of affairs. Roles only have meaning in relationship to other roles. The distinction between roles and actions is that roles define *what* has to be done rather than *how* it should be done. As such we regard roles as an abstraction away from actions. Actions are defined as operations that change or maintain the state of the system or affect the outside world.

3.3 The Basic Types of Structural Relationships

The peer and power relationships may be viewed as relationships at different ends of a co-worker relationship spectrum. Thus a total power relationship is where one agent is totally subservient to another agent, and a total peer relationship is where neither agent is subservient in any way to the other agent. There are of course an infinite number of possible relationships in the middle. The difference between a power / peer relationship and a service relationship is that power / peer relationships tend to exist within organisational boundaries, where as service relationships tend to cross organisational boundaries.

3.4 Power Relationships

The essence of a power relationship is that one agency has the power to make and enforce demands on another agency. It is important to note however that the enforcement of these demands may be made via a third agency. An example of a power relationship is the *supervisor-subordinate* relationship that can exist in most organisations, there are however, many different types of this relationship. In this relationship the supervisor has the power to define the responsibilities and obligations that a subordinate is required to fulfil, and to judge whether or not the responsibilities were correctly discharged.

The subordinate is not totally subservient to the supervisor in that the responsibilities and obligations that the subordinate is required to fulfil are defined by means of interaction between the two agencies. The types of power relationships that can exist between two agencies within an organisation can be defined with reference to the types of interactions that are meaningful for the two agencies to engage in. For example if a person's boss punishes them and they think that the punishment was unfair then they may appeal to a higher authority, the final authority being, of course, the law courts. The nature of these relationships is very complex and something that the problem solver would need to explore carefully and in depth with the problem owners.

3.5 Peer Relationships

The peer relationship is a far more subtle relationship than the power relationship as this relationship appears to be more social in nature than the power relationship. The nature of a peer relationship is that of equality. In a peer relationship there is no implication of enforcement, in fact, it is exactly the lack of this attribute that is characteristic of peer relationships and makes them special. Thus when two agents are in this relationship they may request that each other perform various tasks, however they lack the facility to enforce execution. Hence agreements to perform actions are achieved by means of mutual agreement.

3.6 Service Relationships

In a service relationship one or both of the agents have the power to invoke the execution of a predefined and agreed task by another agent. This task will in some way relate to both the invoking and executing agents. The difference between a service relationship and a power relationship is that when the consuming agent is dissatisfied with the service provided by the supplying agent then the consuming agent may appeal to a third agent. It is this third agent that has the ability to enforce its judgements on both the supplying and consuming agents. A service relationship is in essence one agent invoking the performance of a predefined task by another agent with predefined rules for the enforcement of the correct execution of that task.

Consumer–Supplier - The nature of the consumer–supplier contractual relationship is one of a supplier delivering a predetermined service at the request of a consumer. The nature of the predetermined service that the supplier is required to deliver is something that is established via a negotiation process. This process is something that both the supplier and the consumer are required to have been engaged in prior to the service invocation. The key to understanding this relationship is in understanding that the service is requested by the consumer. The easiest way to illustrate the meaning of this relationship is with an example. A householder has purchases a washing machine from the regional electricity board, as a direct result of which a one year contractual service relationship is established with the board. The nature of the contractual service relationship is one that is defined and enforced by today's legal system. If the washing machine malfunctions in any way the householder may invoke the service relationship by engaging in a conversation with the regional electricity board. The purpose of this conversation is to arrange for the malfunctioning washing machine to be fixed. The regional electricity board is bound by the contractual relationship to arrange for the washing machine to be repaired in a timely manner. If the househlder is dissatisfied with the performance of the regional electricity board in any way then he/she may appeal to the legal system for satisfaction.

Client–Server - In the client–server contractual relationship both parties may engage in the process of service invocation. The client may invoke a service supplied by the server and the server may offer the service to the client without a prior service invocation from the client. The contractual relationship is used to define not only the nature of the service but also the conditions under which that service may be invoked by the client and offered by the server. An example of such a system is a client server computer system where the client is using a password service that is managed and maintained by the server. Thus the client may request that their copy of the passwords be updated. or the server may force the client to update his/her copy of the passwords.

Consumer–Provider - In the consumer–provider contractual relationship the provider undertakes to provide a service to the consumer, in addition the role of service invoker is something that is performed by the provider. Thus we may say that the consumer–provider contractual relationship is the exact opposite of the consumer–supplier contractual relationship. The consumer–provider contractual relationship is used to define not only the nature of the service but also the conditions under which that service may be invoked by the provider and used by the consumer. A simple example of this relationship is that of marriage, as in the marriage contractual relationship the husband undertakes to provide for his wife, and vice versa. The conditions that are placed on this service are that it shall be provided in sickness and in health.

Customer–Supplier - The nature of the customer–supplier contractual relationship is one of either party being able to engage in a conversation with the other party. The purpose of this conversation is to establish another contractual relationship along with the rules governing its existence and meaningfulness. In addition, the nature of the conversation that both parties may engage in is one of negotiation. An example of the customer supplier contractual relationship is one of salesperson–customer. In this relationship the purpose of the conversation is to purchase an item and thereby establish a contractual relationship. This relationship is one that society as a whole defines and consequently the legal system is required to monitor and enforce it. The legal system has over the years established vast volumes of law relating to the governing of this type of relationship. These guidelines govern such things as the permissible and meaningful behaviour of parties that are currently engaged in the relationship. In addition, they also govern the meaningfulness of any contractual relationships that are established as a direct result of this relationship.

4.0 Enterprise Modelling

I have chosen to illustrate our ideas by means of an example from the medical domain which I have been investigating. Figure 2 represents a hospital's view of how the medical encounter currently looks. It should be pointed out that all the agents depicted in Figure 2 represent human agents. In Figure 2 the agencies involved are depicted as rectangles. The responsibility relationships between agencies are depicted as thick double lines. The rectangles within reactangles shown in Figure 3 and 4 represent the roles and services that a agent performs in order to fulfill a responsibility. Roles are linked together by means of a responsibility relationship. The responsibility relationship and its associated roles and services are a shorthand for the framework that gives meaning and defines and interactions through the agents communicate and fulfill their responsibilities. The responsibility relationships allow us to identify the resources that mediate that relationship. For example, in Figure 3 we can observe that the responsibility relationship between the *sick person* agent and the *administering* agent is mediated by the resource *medication*.

In the following section, a brief description of the decomposition of a health care delivery agent is presented. In this representation. both the structural roles (such as Client–Server and Carer–Ward) and the resources through which interaction takes place are represented in the same diagram.

Central to the concept of health care delivery are the role and responsibilities of the physician as embodied in the western medical tradition. It is clear from the assertions made about this role that several agencies are involved:

- The *diagnosing agent*, who obtains data and specimens from the sick person and interprets them in terms of symptoms. The context for this activity is the Doctor—Patient relationship (in the strict sense). The diagnosing agent produces a diagnosis and a statement of requirements on the treatment in terms of the medicinal effect which is required. This is presented to the prescribing agent in a peer/colleague relationship. To be effective in delivering health care, these agents, together with the counselling agent, must act as a team if they are not composed into the role of a single person. The diagnosing agent is required to make all the data gathered and utilised in making a diagnosis available to the administering agent. The reason for this is that under law the administering agent is responsible for the effects that the medication has on the sick person.

- The *prescribing agent*, who acts on the basis of the diagnosis and requirements and produces a prescription which has some authentication token attached. Since this information is interpreted in the context of a client server relationship, there is a requirement for some mechanism which will ensure that the prescription is not only appropriate but also available for dispensing.

- The *dispensing agent*, who shares some of the responsibility for the appropriateness of the medication. There is a requirement that medication should only be dispensed in accordance with the code defining appropriate dosage and application. If, as in the case of the U.S. mental health system, the anonymity of the patient must be protected from the pharmacist, then the prescription must be presented with a coded identity. In order to discharge the obligations of the dispensing agent, the pharmacist must have access to the medical records but only by means and in terms of these codes. In U.K. primary health care, it is part of the G.P.—Pharmacist—Community relationship that the dispensing agent will know or find out sufficient information about the patient to exercise this checking function. This contrasts with the case of venereal disease where the dispensing agent and the dispensary information is internal to the clinic. It represents a closed information domain in order to protect the patient's interests in confidentiality and thus minimise the risk of treatment avoidance and its social consequences. The dispensing agent allocates medication which is both material and information (in the case of drugs). The original source indicates a rule that an independent dispensing record must be made by the dispensing agent.

- The *administering agent*, who administers the treatment according to the instructions of the prescription. Since, in principle, the anonymity of the patient cannot be preserved with respect to the nursing agent, it is clear that if it is required with respect to the pharmacist, then the nursing agent must have appropriate access to the medical records to decode the identity of the patient. A surgeon discharges administering agency as does a nurse; at this stage we do not distinguish between them. The hospital has a legal requirement placed upon it that the administering agent is responsible for the effects that the medication has on the sick person.

- The *counselling agent* is the agent who has the obligation to inform the civil person of all the information judged to be necessary and appropriate concerning the health care being given. It is on the basis of this information that informed consent can be given.

- The *client agent* is the agent who in the case of a public health enterprise is the individual who is being informed of health hazards. In the case of health care, it is the individual who requests treatment.

- The *civil person*, who is the individual who has the right to be kept appropriately informed and who exercises the civil and legal rights of the sick person in the context of the medical environment. In the case of a baby, this would be the parents or guardian; in the case of a mentally ill person it could be the next of kin or the civil authority. The usual case is for the civil and the sick person to be the same individual.

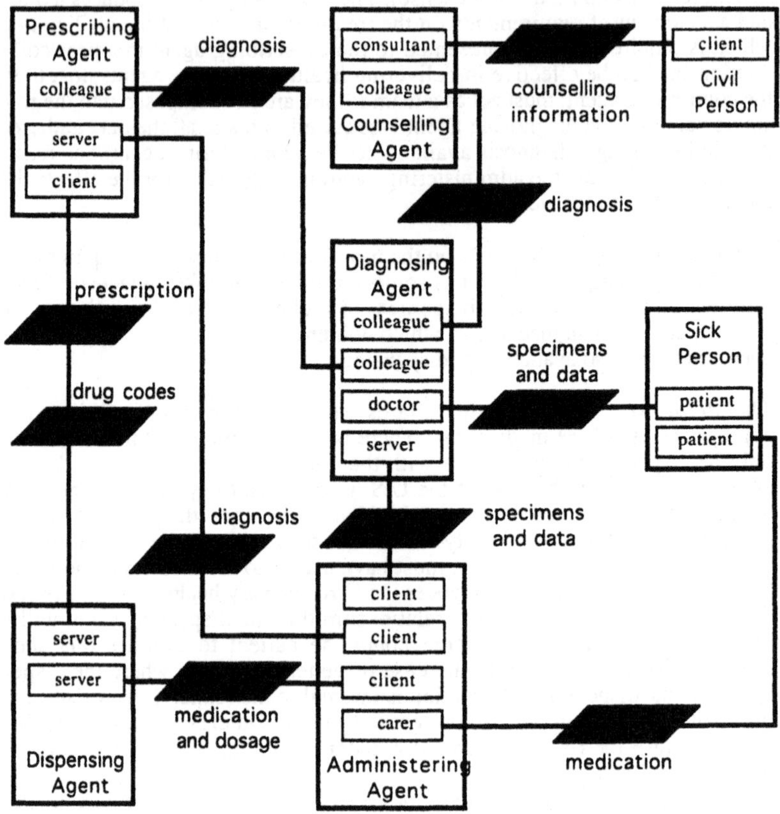

Figure 2 The Current Health Care Enterprise

The hospital from which this case study was taken was looking to replace the human agent which administers drugs with a computer based agent. The hospital believed that this would decrease the chance of human error, with regard to the correct drugs being administered, and would free up the nurses time so that they could concentrate on the human side of caring for a patient. The two questions that management wanted to answer were:

- What implication does adoption of computer based administering agents have on the organisation's responsibility ?

- How does the organisation need to re-align its work-flows and responsibilities so as to fulfill its organisational responsibilities ?

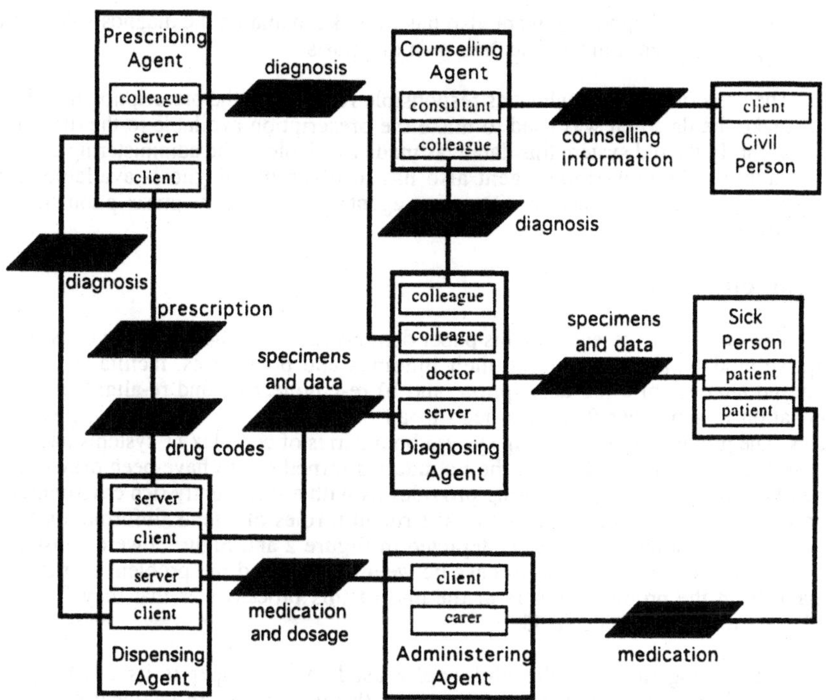

Figure 3 The Proposed Health Care Enterprise

Figure 3 represents the re-structuring and re-alignment of the organisation with regards to the adoption and utilisation of an automated administering agent. The above diagram represents the re-assignment and re-alignment of several key organisational responsibilities. There are several points about Figure 3 that should be noted.

- The administering agent has become an automaton. This agent can no longer be held responsible for the effects that a medication has on a patient. For this reason all of the information that the administering agent requires in order to make an informed decision as to whether or not to administer the drug has moved to the dispensing agent. Under the new system the dispensing agent is responsible for the actions and effects of the administering agent.

- The dispensing agent now has to make an informed decision whether or not the prescription and diagnosis is correct. In order to make this decision the dispensing agent needs access to the diagnosis and medical history data. In the current system (See Figure 2) the dispensing agent is the pharmacy and the current pharmacy does not have experience at making medical decisions. Consequently if the new system is to be adopted then the pharmacy will have to be trained and given the skills to make the key medical decisions. In addition, the hospital also now has to prove that the administering agent was told to administer the correct medication. From Figure 3 we can identify the resource flow between the dispensing agent and the administering agent, and we can ask the following question: "What type of resource flows between the agents and who has access to this resource ?"

- The diagnosing agent who was responsible for performing the diagnosis now has to make the data that was used to make the diagnosis available to the dispensing agent. In the old system this data was made available to the administering agent. In addition, the diagnosing agent also has to make available the diagnosis so that the dispensing agent can validate their own diagnosis.

- The prescribing agent who was responsible for making the prescription now has to make the data that was used to make the prescription available to the dispensing agent. In the old system this data was made available to the administering agent. In addition, the prescribing agent also has to make the diagnosis available to the dispensing agent so that the dispensing agent can validate the prescription and drug codes.

5.0 Conclusions

The case study presented in this paper demonstrates that the process of constructing enterprise models, and determining their bindings and boundaries, facilitates in the a) design and analysis of a job description, and b) re-engineering and re-alignment of the organisation in a manner that pays heed to an organisation's requirements, goals, and policies. The problem of determining system boundaries of complex IT systems has meant that mistakes have occurred where the boundaries turned out to have been drawn in the wrong place. Responsibility modelling provides us with a sufficiently rich environment in which we can represent the organisational structure, roles of agents, information flows, and resource utilisation. The models depicted in Figure 2 and Figure 3 were constructed through a dialectic and iterative process between myself and the problem owners. The feedback from the problem owners at the end of this process was that they found the models easy to use and understand.

The driving thrust of the philosophy used in this paper is its advocation of involving policy makers and problem owners throughout the re-engineering and re-alignment process. It is a process of shifting the balance of responsibility between system owner and system designer away from the 'owner states, designer solves' model towards a relationship in which the problem owner helps the problem solver understand the problem, and the problem solver helps the problem owner understand the implications of possible solutions. By involving the policy makers and problem owners in the re-design process and focusing upon policies we can have greater confidence that the re-engineered organisation still adheres to its policies.

To sum up, responsibility modelling recognises that the re-alignment of organisations with regard to confidentiality, safety and security policies is best accomplished by a technique that combines the social aspects of a system with the technical, and adheres to the principle of giving the customer what the customer needs and not what the system designers think the customer wants.

6.0 References

[1] T. Winograd. F. Flores, Understanding Computers and Cognition. Addison-Wesley, 1987

[2] M. Banton, Role: An Introduction to the Study of Social Relations. Tavistock, 1965.

[3] K. Lyytinen and R.A. Hirscheim, "*Information Systems Failures: A Survey and Classification of Empirical Literature*", Oxford Surveys in Information Technology, Vol 4, pp. 257 - 309, 1987.

[4] P. Beynon-Davies, (1995), Information Systems 'Failure': The Case of the London Ambulance Service's Computer Aided Despatch Project, European Journal of Information Systems, Vol 4, pp. 171-184

[5] M. S. Bogner, Human Errors in Medicine, Lawrence Erlbaum Associates, 1994.

[6] P. Checkland, Systems Thinking, Systems Practice, Wiley, 1986.

[7] Joyce Glasser, Organisational Aspects of System Failure: A Case Study at the Los Angeles Police Department, Proceedings of the 2nd International Conference on Information Systems, pp. 233-245, 1981.

[8] Stephen Sloane,The use of Artificial Intelligence by the United States Navy: Case Study of a Failure, AI Magazine, Spring, pp. 80 - 92, 1991.

[9] M. Lynne Markus, (1983), Power, politics and MIS Implementation, Communications of the ACM, 26(6), pp. 430 - 444.

[10] Dan Bernard, (1979), Management Issues in Co-operative Computing, ACM Computing Surveys, 11(1), pp. 3 - 17

[11] R. C. Barrows and P. D. Clayton, Privacy, Confidentiality and Electronic Medical Records, Journal of the American Medical Informatics Association, 3(2), pp. 139 - 148, 1996.

[12] Audit Commission, For Your Information: A Study of Information Management and Systems in the Acute Hospital, Her Majesty's Stationary Office (HMSO), 1995.

[13] R. Fox, "*No Laughing Matter*", Communications of the ACM, 38(5),pp. 10, 1995.

[14] N. Leveson, Safeware: System Safety and Computers, Adison-Wesley, 1995.

[15] Kling, R. "*Social Analyses of Computing: Theoretical Perspectives in Recent Empirical Research*", ACM Computing Surveys, 12(1), pp. 61 - 110, 1980.

[16] David Harvey, Re-Engineering - The Critical Success Factors, Business Intelligence, 1995.

Keeping Confidence in Confidentiality: Linking Ethics, Efficacy, and Opportunity in Health Care Computing - A Case Study

Michael Rigby

Lecturer in Health Planning and Management

Centre for Health Planning and Management, Darwin Building, Keele University, Keele, Staffordshire, ST5 5BG, U.K.

"We are all in the gutter, but some of us are looking at the stars."
Oscar Wilde [1]

Summary

The application of computing technology to healthcare is long-established and rapidly growing, with new horizons opening up rapidly as a result of increased processing power, lower costs, increased recognition of the potential improvements to health care and its delivery, and the managerial and research potential of quality databases capable of easier analysis. However, new technical opportunities often need matching new policies and controls, and this has not had sufficient attention.

In early 1996 in England the National Health Service Executive applied policy pressures to maximise certain benefits from a planned information technology infrastructure[2]. Unfortunately, this expedition of specific applications ahead of deliberation of all the issues moved the overdue debate into crisis rather than constructive mode, and it thus now forms a valuable if unfortunate case study for other countries on the importance of gaining evidence-based round table consensus on the matching benefits and controls for innovation, at policy and practice level, ahead of general implementation. This paper summarises issues that have arisen; identifies weaknesses in the immediate professional response to a policy vacuum; and suggests the foundations for a more soundly-based approach.

Introduction

As health care is concerned with services to patients and populations, it is appropriate that a major focus in healthcare computing developments should be on personal health records as the basic units of holding information. However, the drive for exploitation of information processing power has not been matched by consideration of how the technological opportunities also raise new ethical and professional issues. This has caused replication of the cycle which is so familiar from watching the devolved roll-out of other new health technologies - namely euphoria; unanticipated problems; perceived crisis; public recrimination; belated rational discussion; and finally, overdue agreement on sound controls - as seen, for instance, with the advent of minimally-invasive surgery[3].

Neither public confidence, ethics, science, nor the technology concerned are well served by the kind of acrimonious arguments exchanged in the mass media, the computing press, or the conference platform in a campaign which seemed more about winning than proving appropriateness or effectiveness of planned security controls over new technological applications. There has been even less attempt to exploit the potential of the new information technology to address security weaknesses of traditional paper records, or to create new sophistication of confidentiality hierarchies. Anxieties are further raised when the key paper in the scientific medical literature proposing new solutions opened by citing items from the popular press which have no proven link with computer applications (and indeed are problems which could more likely have been prevented by good computer-based security)[4].

Unfortunately, as aptly phrased by Oscar Wilde, no party comes out looking immaculate, yet all claimed to see the true light - an inevitable risk of urgent retrospective policy making under conflicting pressures. This case study demonstrates the importance of dispassionately injecting understanding, fact, principle, and realism into a fundamental topic at the formative stage of strategy. Only in this way can one seek the timeless pure light from the heavens, as opposed to the stars before the eyes seen following the upper-cut to the jaw.

Background

For over three decades computers have been used in health care, not least to hold and process aspects of individuals' records. Applications in the U.K. have developed separately in the very different domains of primary care, community care, and secondary care. In some areas, such as pathology and radiology, it would now be difficult for clinicians to deliver effective care without them. In other areas, too, such as primary care, they have become endemic and part of the culture of good practice [5]. There have to date been few complaints of misuse, itself arguably surprising given the scale of the National Health Service (NHS), though this is no ground for complacency. The British Medical Association (BMA) itself is a strong proponent of effective use of information in clinical practice, as is shown from choosing the title "The Heart of the Matter - The Vital Role of Information in Clinical Practice" for its first international conference on the topic.

Strategy or Straight Jacket?

However, piecemeal development of healthcare computing is unlikely to be the best way forward. Lack of standards (of data items, of information, of technical inter-connections, or of clinician inter-face) can only lead to fragmentation, waste, and risk of error. Leaving a supplier market to identify best solutions is likely to lead to expensive mistakes and blind alleys on the one hand, and to potentially monopolistic situations on the other. In particular, it is a fraught way of developing necessary standards - of practice, of data, and of technology. Thus the central co-ordination of a development and evaluation programme, but with results in the public domain so as to give market freedom to optimise applications, is inherently justifiable on grounds of public interest and efficiency, and therefore of ethics, as well as acting as a catalyst for scientific developments. Hence the appropriateness in principle of an Information Strategy, a need which was intended to be met by the aforementioned Information Management and Technology Strategy[2] insofar as England is concerned.

This strategy has a vision of enabling clinicians to deliver good care by improving their use of clinical information, both person-based and knowledge-based. It also has an element of national standard information handling infrastructure to seek accuracy and cost-effectiveness in the management of the health care system. Again this is desirable *per se*, and seeks to build on principles which have served the NHS well, such as common general practitioner registration and service claims systems through standard Family Health Service Authority (FHSA) software applications (including development of paperless interfaces with practice computers).

This duality of objective, though, has laid the foundation for current differences of priorities and values, enhanced by a perceived ambiguity as to whether central interests in the NHS and Government are seeking to empower clinicians and provider organisations through better use of information, or to control the NHS and indeed regulate society. Thus the central policy and coordination aspects can also be a threat, in terms both of how policy is determined and in the priorities and timescales for implementation

Specific to the themes of confidentiality and security of personal records, this has led to claim and counter-claim about perceptions of enablement or impedance; irresponsibility or protectionism; rashness or Ludditism; empowerment or subversion; and informed decision making or centralist power. Above all in the context of this paper, differences of approach have arisen over perceptions of short-termism jeopardising confidence building; and of supposed public interest jeopardising confidentiality. Clearly, this has done nothing to advance the patient's or clinician's interests in improved application healthcare computing, and is an important lesson on how not to develop the ethical and control aspects of harnessing the developing technology.

Of Eagles and Ostriches

However, this situation could not have occurred if so many parties had not been lacking in their responsibilities to provide a lead in openly addressing the public and professional ethical issues. Current tensions can only be addressed effectively if their context is understood. Where clear high-level vision, scanning the landscape for the best routes forward, could reasonably have been expected, at best there was a much more terrestrial and immediate viewpoint. By way of explanation not recrimination, the following can be cited as key examples:

- Failure by the NHS Executive's Information Management Group to put emphasis on seeking integrated multi-professional views to shape, prioritise, or lead the overall English strategy[6,7].
- Lack of any attempt by the health professions to come together jointly to develop a view or vision[7], notwithstanding recognition of the pivotal role of information in clinical practice, and the centrally recognised value of groups such as the Strategic Advisory Group on Nursing Information Systems (SAGNIS).
- Pressure by the Information Management Group to achieve rapid progress with components of the Strategy, rather than address important issues raised in the process[8].
- Prolonged delay by the Department of Health in issuing definitive and acceptable long-promised guidelines on confidentiality[9], when they were greatly needed to precede and thus shape strategic issues.
- Inadequacy in some respects of the Department of Health Guidelines when issued[10], in particular their reliance upon the common law concept of duty of confidence and upon implied consent, neither of which has been adequately tested in court of law in health record contexts.

- Failure of professional bodies to follow through informatics issues identified in professional studies, as for instance with the Royal College of Psychiatrists' important study the current state and future potential of electronic record systems in psychiatry[11].
- General low priority given to confidentiality and security by many hospitals, as identified by the Audit Commission, in regards to paper records but potentially also with computerised records[12].
- A perceived concentration by the Information Management Centre arm of the Information Management Group upon security of electronic systems against physical threats which, whilst vitally important and under-appreciated, are only part of the potential threat. However, the co-director has recently published a clear and dispassionate overview of the issues and principal stakeholder positions, with a patient focus[13].
- A reluctance by leading professional journals to publish papers considering confidentiality and security, even following positive refereeing, unless they can demonstrate empirically that the principles described have actually reduced breaches of confidentiality[14].

A Spark for the Tinder

Into this dry and flammable tinder box came the inevitable inflammatory spark. This happened to be the NHS Network, intended to be a means of allowing confidential data to be transmitted within the NHS in a secure environment. Its main predecessor was Healthlink, a private NHS network linking FHSAs, and more latterly general practitioners, which has generally been found to be beneficial not least to general practitioners in reducing paperwork and increasing speed and accuracy. Unfortunately, between mention as part of the Strategy and publication of the full project specification, the NHS Executive view of the Network changed from a means for the NHS to transmit messages, into a network which would enable remote interrogation of a clinical information system outside the control of the record custodians. Not surprisingly, this led to major anxieties, with the BMA stepping into the unfilled role of defender of the ethics.

Apart from the issue of whether the NHS and its professions ever wanted this new functionality, the main themes in an uncomfortable debate have been -

- whether and how personal data sent on the network should be encrypted to protect against unauthorised interception and subsequent misuse;
- the appropriateness of the risk model used;
- the security of the systems linked to, and thus by the new definition interlinked by, the network;
- adequacy of the control mechanisms for the network and its connected end user systems;

- clearing houses for contract and activity data, their controls, and their scope to further process personal data, the source data for which must (by national policy directive) in future be supplied by means of the network;
- an apparent potential for the Executive to use the interrogative facility to access clinical systems on grounds of monitoring performance or resources.

All these are serious points, but are outside the scope of this paper. They merely emphasise the importance of there being advance discussion and agreement between policy makers and professional bodies on policy and purpose, if there is to be mutual (and public) confidence in sophisticated computer and telecommunications applications. However, the focus of this paper will be upon returning to what should always have been the starting point, namely the confidentiality of the personal health record and its core purpose of enabling the individual citizen to receive good quality, timely health care. Unfortunately, but understandably given the time constraints, the BMA response itself confused the secondary and the primary issues.

As well as seeking to have the above network-related points addressed, the BMA also sought to ensure that clinical computer systems which would in future be interlinked by the network were in fact secure enough for this (despite the fact that it would have been a better strategy to challenge more robustly the interrogative aspect of the network, at least for the early stages.) Recognising that the Department of Health confidentiality guidance was then still awaited, and that there was limited professionally-backed guidance on what constituted a safe computer system, in January 1996 the BMA published a consultation document entitled "Security in Clinical Information Systems"[15].

The Blue Light Syndrome

However, in seeking to prevent a conflagration, the BMA response engendered the common uncertainty which follows the noise and bustle of any emergency service mobilisation, concerning the balance between control, prevention, and education. In particular, two areas of confusion have resulted.

First, the BMA document appeared in the same week as a British Medical Journal (BMJ) item of similar title[4]. However, whilst the BMJ paper opened with the references from the popular press to the general availability of medical records for financial considerations, the consultation document opened with reference to the NHS network. As both items postulated the same set of nine new principles for protection of personal information, it was not clear which threat they were seeking to address, save that they appeared to have been conceived as a defensive measure against threats, rather than as a positive iteration of the rights of the citizen.

Secondly, external confusion has been caused by the fact that the BMA document contained only minimal reference to consultation (the only mention being in the fifth paragraph of the Foreword), and there was no reference to any process for a debate. It was thus not surprising that many assumed the consultationto be cursory, and that the principles have been imposed by the medical profession *de facto*, a position created more by default than by intention.

Finally, the strident nature of the network encryption debate has discouraged more reflective analysis. For instance, the Health directorates of the other three home countries of the United Kingdom have stood back from discussion even though the BMA principles would, by definition, apply also to them. It appears they were reluctant "to move into the logically sound position in the middle ground, as that would simply mean getting caught in the broadsides of between the entrenched positions of the two factions" [16]. A similar position has also apparently been adopted by at least one Royal College, even though it sees problems for good care delivery presented by the BMA proposals[17].

<u>The Policy Lesson</u>

The lesson from this part of the case study is the importance of agreeing at an early stage the person-based, public, and professional values, information system objectives, and enforceable safeguards. By waiting until a real issue arises, the differing perceptions of viewpoint and intention are ingrained, and therefore the situation analysis becomes clouded by orientational as well as empirical interpretations. Consequently, time, resources, and above all trust, are lost - to the detriment of all interests. This learning point is generic to all areas of processing of personal information, and is not unique to health care.

Consideration of the BMA Document

Given that the BMA document[15] has created a major impact within the United Kingdom and abroad, this paper will now consider its practical, technical, and ethical dimensions before moving on to postulate alternative approaches. It is pivotal in the English NHS policy debate, though by implication it applies to the whole of the United Kingdom, but coming from an internationally respected medical body which advocates evidence-based medicine it should also be seminally robust. Though relating entirely to health care, as this is one of the most sensitive areas of personal information it should be a valuable learning ground for other application domains.

Testing the Premise

If confidence truly is to be achieved by confidentiality principles, a more robust debate than is currently taking place is needed. In fact, the document shows the difficulty of moving in haste into poorly charted waters. Probably because of the extension from technical security issues to confidentiality of clinical information and how it is handled, it does not stand up well to detailed scrutiny in the latter domain. The principle problems are identified below:-

- **Security Model or Organisational Methods?:** The document correctly states that a security policy provides protection, and is driven by a threat model (identifying what malicious or accidental disasters might occur). However, the document goes on to propose radical changes to operational practice within the NHS, without directly mapping these proposals to the threat model, and sets out principles which would impede current good clinical practice. This is far more than a security model.
- **Security or Confidentiality?:** Confidentiality and Security must be distinguished. Security is a technical process - it seeks to take all feasible, affordable, and acceptable steps to protect a defined position with regard to information collection, storage, and transmission. It is not concerned with the processing and use *per se* of the information, only with whether this has been authorised. Confidentiality is the boundary within which the data subject expects their data to be used; it is that which security measures seek to protect, and is based on personal values (and is therefore a mix of generic or societal values and the values of each individual person - presenting particular ethical and practical challenges). The document covers far more than security - it proposes new principles of confidentiality and clinical practice, and if this is necessary it should be titled, presented and reviewed as such.
- **Absence of Goal Definition:** In seeking to redress a weakness (in this case the weaknesses of paper records and the potential for abuse of electronic records), three alternative standards can be postulated - better than the current situation (even if by a modest amount); a specified acceptable and achievable explicit set of performance standards (including numeric ranges); or perfection. The document states (page 1) that "security of electronic records must meet or exceed the standard that should be applied to paper records", but then goes on to propose principles which imply a demand for perfection. Costs, justification, and expectation will be very different according to alternative aspiration.
- **Lack of Balanced Evidence:** The development of policy should be based on impartial review of the literature and empirical evidence. However, while the BMA document cites press reports evidence of apparent misuse of computer records, it quotes none of the evidence of the benefits to patients of automated records, even though a solid body of scientific literature is

building up in the United States[18,19]. In the UK the first proof of benefits in community health was published twenty years ago[20], and the recent analysis of evidence from primary care is also positive[21], while the Audit Commission[12] has cogently argued the benefits to patients which are waiting to be gained through hospital systems. Also in the UK, benefits realisation methodologies have been developed by health professionals to identify and achieve intended net patient benefits[22], while at European level a special study has addressed the value of health telematics in pursuing the twin goals of equity and quality[23], including British achievements in community care[24]. Further, the BMA document indicates (on page 7) that about one electronic message in 10,000 will become corrupted, without any balancing estimate of the number of potentially harmful errors of entry or interpretation which occur in handwritten clinical records.

- **Security Culture:** Many see it as important to enhance security by all possible steps - a *kaizan* approach, for instance replacing names and plain language diagnosis on audit and contracting documents, where some form of patient identifier is necessary but not full identification, or use of reference numbers on specimens. This does not pretend to be total anonymity, but does reduce the chance of casual accidental browsing, and of a staff member realising they are handling material related to a relative or acquaintance. However, the document dismissively misrepresents this as a false attempt at full anonymity, which is not the intention, thereby undermining the importance of a attempts to create a security-thinking culture.
- **Risk Analysis:** There is a recognised science, and specific quantification methodologies, to identify risk. The BMA has identified the principle source of risk as being internal, but has not sought in a structured way to break down and quantify this. Thus an important methodology, and potential supporting evidence, has been ignored.
- **Value Based or System Based?:** The approach adopted seeks to put forward an organisational framework, based on procedures focused on the professional provider of services. The values or views of the individual client cannot readily be accommodated.
- **Support the Business Objectives:** It is self-evident that security principles should support and protect the organisation's core business objectives, and above all thereby ensure the interests of the personal consumer are well met. The document demonstrates the difficulties of using a technical approach in isolation, and in haste, in a complex area such as health care. The following are examples of ways in which important areas or practitioners in health care will find the document unsatisfactory:

  Abuses the concept of "Need-to-Know": A frequent approach to defining the right to information about a patient is the "need-to-know", and very specifically this is the information requirement corollary of the clinician's "duty of care". Need-to-know is thus a valid clinical test, but the document dismisses it as "administrative convenience", which totally destroys its intent and value.

Misrepresents Clinical Practice: The document states (pages 11 and 22) that normal clinical practice is for records to be clinician-based rather than patient-based. This totally misrepresents the hospital patient record and clinical practice, and goes against both Government policy and best professional practice for integrated care, particularly in mental health and community care. Profession-specific records may complement the main record, but an integrated prime record must exist.

Stigmatises Mental Health: The document lists psychiatric history as *prima facie* highly sensitive, but the recording of conditions such as Alzheimer's Disease is important and no disgrace, and less sensitive than recording the temporary address for a woman seeking refuge from marital violence. It is important in a professional document that a more enlightened attitude to mental health should prevail, seeking to remove the stigma rather than render the clinical facts ultra-secret, and thus *ipso facto* outside the discussion though controlled by it.

Informed Consent: The document puts understandable emphasis on personal consent. In health care this is a difficult area under many circumstances. First, by definition at the onset of hospitalising illness, the patient is anxious even if not distressed or comatose. Secondly, it could be submitted that they only consented at the time in order not to upset the doctor or to delay treatment. Thirdly, it could be argued that consent was not informed as the person would need to understand the full working of a hospital far beyond the consulting room or bedside, when in fact patients expect hospitals to know their business of how to get on with providing sound, effective, and quality monitored treatment using the full clinical record. Fourthly, children, the frail elderly, persons with mental illness or learning disabilities, and those with poor English, will be further disadvantaged.

Practicality: Proposals must be practical if they are to be achieved, whilst recognising the risk of this being used as an excuse not to implement change. However, a parallel paper identifies with empirical evidence the difficulties the document's proposals would create in a typical general hospital [25].

Anti-Managerial: Any healthcare system has to be managed, though this itself raises ethical issues which need further debate. The document makes no mention of service management, but does refer several times to administrators in disparaging connotations. This is not a realistic, responsible, nor tenable approach.

- **Completeness:** Security, confidentiality, and ethics are all complex issues with many aspects. It is important to define the areas to be addressed, then to cover these completely, otherwise important issues will be assumed unimportant. Despite its title, in security terms the document is incomplete, as it only considers the technical aspects of computer access and network protection. There are many other aspects of data security, including physical protection, which are very different from paper record security, with some enhanced risks, but also with new opportunities such as separate site back-up duplication of the entire record sets. These important aspects are not covered. The simultaneous BMJ paper well covered some, but not all, of these.

- **Justification:** The document fails its own test. It states (on page 23) that "the onus is on the proposers of 'patient-based' record systems to provide a clear statement of the expected health gains and analyse the threats, the cost of added countermeasures and the likely effects of the residual risk". This is a sound principle which should apply to all healthcare developments, whether technological or process. As indicated above, work in this direction with regard to computer-held patient records has been ignored in producing the document. More importantly, that very test is not applied within the document itself in regard to the nine new principles it promulgates, nor their financial and human resource costs.

Testing the Principles

The document's most creative aspect is the putting forward of nine new security principles to constitute a Security Policy for personal health data, as part of an identified need for a new paradigm for personal records. It is appreciated that the models for military and financial applications do not serve personal records well. In fact, the proposed new concepts are confidentiality as much as security topics, and themselves do not hold up well against the needs and patient interests of healthcare other than possibly in primary care. Though the innovative intent is surely to be welcomed, reflective analysis shows the following problems:

Principles or Rules?: A principle is "a fundamental truth" [26]. Truths and values should indeed be the building blocks of confidentiality policies, which should then be protected by security policies. What are put forward in the BMA document are operational Rules, which are the means by which Principles are implemented. They are essential in their own right, but need Principles to precede them to give the value framework. This confusion between Rules and Principles is the cause of much of the concern created by the BMA document, and a key point to be understood in the development means of protecting personal information.

Principle 1: "Each identifiable clinical record shall be marked with an access control list naming the people or groups of people who read it and append data to it. The system shall prevent anyone not on the access control list from accessing the record in any way." This fits well with primary care. However, in hospital care either the patient attends as an emergency, or else they are referred by a clinician and the computer record created at that stage. There will be particular problems of informed consent. This proposal would also create additional systems and paperwork, which by definition will fall to health professionals to administer in the clinical setting.

Principle 2: "A clinician may open a record with herself and the patient on the access control list. Where a patient has been referred, she may open a record with herself, the patient, and the referring clinician(s) on the access control list." This is seriously flawed. It disenfranchises the patient by being clinician, not patient, focused. It suggests opening the record ahead of determining the patient's wishes. In particular, the patient may not want the referring clinician to have access to the record's detail; indeed, that may have been a reason for the patient seeking a referral.

Principle 3: "One of the clinicians on the access control list must be marked as being responsible. Only she may alter the access control list, and she may only add other health care professionals to it." Again, this is seriously impractical. First, it does not allow for the subsequent absence of the "responsible" clinician, as it allows no alternative procedure. Secondly, it does not reflect the subtle but important changes in balance with hospital or community care patients who may have concurrent conditions, which change in relative significance with the passage of time - for instance, when the mild cardiac problem becomes acute while the orthopaedic surgery is healing.

Principle 4: "The responsible clinician must notify the patient of the names on his record's access control list when it is opened, of all subsequent additions, and whenever responsibility is transferred. His consent must also be obtained, except in emergency or in the case of statutory exemptions." The principle of keeping the patient informed is sound; the practicality and cost may be less so, as they are not considered. The wording is unfortunate in giving the record, not the patient, ownership of the access control. It will not overcome the cited example of impersonation if information is then released other than electronically.

Principle 5: "No-one shall have the ability to delete clinical information until the appropriate time period has expired." This is current, and essential, good practice.

Principle 6: "All accesses to clinical records shall be marked on the record with the subject's name, as well as the date and time. An audit trail must also be kept of all deletions." This does not go far enough - there should be a full audit trail of all activity. Audit trails must also be indelible, and capable of interpretation.

Principle 7: "Information derived from record A may be appended to record B if and only if B's access control list is contained in A's." This is seriously flawed as it focuses on the clinician, not the patient.

Principle 8: "There shall be effective measures to prevent the aggregation of personal health information. In particular, patients must receive special notification if any person whom it is proposed to add to their access control list already has access to personal health information on a large number of people." This addresses an important point, but given that it includes records with only reference numbers as identifiers, it challenges the practice of public health, audit, outcomes analysis, and effectiveness studies, where the identifier is needed to follow the treatment history. Moreover, it challenges GP registration and fee reimbursement procedures, health insurance funded treatment, and the United Kingdom internal market. These aspects need further study to balance the patient interest in the effective management and development of good care, protection of professional standards, and probity for use of public funds, with the safeguarding of the person's privacy.

Principle 9: "Computer systems that handle personal health information shall have a subsystem that enforces the above principles in an effective way. Its effectiveness shall be subject to evaluation by independent experts." A security subsystem is vitally important. Means of independent evaluation are to be welcomed, but the effect on small clinician-designed systems, and the custodianship of the accreditation system, both need further consideration.

<u>The Ethics of the Principles</u>

Given, then, that the postulated new principles appear in parts to be welcome, but in detail to produce major new problems, what is their overall ethical position? They appear to fail a number of fundamental tests:

Not Person-Based: It is paradoxical that principles aimed to protect personal privacy are not couched in terms of patients' rights, and their control of their care, but are clinician-focused.

Socially Regressive: The BMA principles are framed in a primary care philosophy, and phrased in terms of adult care. Children, the mentally ill, and other groups who are considered in theory to be priority groups are considered last and incompletely yet again, and with no consideration of the problems as to who best speaks on their behalf, not least in disunited families. The proposals are strongly socially regressive.

Integrated Care: It is national policy, supported by professional bodies, that care should be integrated and "seamless". This requires good communication and confidence. Unfortunately, it does not always work perfectly, and most retrospective enquiries into problems of adverse events in mental health and child abuse in particular have shown failure of communication of facts to be a key issue. This needs careful, sound and progressive handling, but moving to clinician-specific records can only work to the detriment of vulnerable patients in priority services.

Quality Criteria: Maxwell published six key quality criteria in the BMJ in 1984[27], and these have become seminal yardsticks by which to measure quality of services. The criteria are that services or procedures shall be measured by their accessibility, relevance, effectiveness, equity, acceptability, and efficiency and economy, primarily from a social or consumer viewpoint. It is difficult to reconcile the BMA proposed principles to these criteria if one takes effective care for the patient as the objective.

"Whistleblowing": There is general recognition that not all health professionals and other employees behave perfectly. There has been increasing concern that staff are discouraged from reporting suspicions. One of the key sources of information to verify or disprove bad practice is the patient record, and particularly items such as times of procedures and drug doses. A prime concern identified in several retrospective enquiries is that early, informal suspicions were not followed up soon enough - yet in a real world most suspicions will be unfounded, but must be investigated to find genuine problems. The BMA principles would require that any senior clinician investigating an allegation or anomaly would have to be declared to every patient whose care was checked as an addition to the access control list, and if possible for their consent to be obtained for this investigative use of records. In the great majority of cases this will raise unnecessary anxieties, and possibly stimulate opportunistic compensation claims, and therefore providers would be even more reluctant to follow up initial intimations of miscondict. Of course, it is important that patients are told if there is a proven possibility that they have been treated with less than competent standards, but the investigatory process itself should not be discouraged.

Public Health and Health Care Development: Little thought is given in the document to discharge of public health requirements, nor to outcomes studies. This needs much more detailed consideration to ensure that longer-term patient interests are not being jeopardised.

Patient Support: The document only quotes one survey of patient opinion, from primary care. Before such radical proposals are instigated universally, it would be essential to obtain public opinion about them and their likely effects.

Those working in the NHS are well aware of patient annoyance that information is not better communicated between clinicians.

Cost Benefit: There is no analysis of the cost (including clinician time) which would be involved. The access control consent procedures would be reminiscent of the procedures once brought in to prevent alleged abuse of the NHS by non-British nationals, whereby a detailed algorithm was designed and every non-emergency patient had to be assessed at the point of first contact. This was a major annoyance to clinicians and to many patients, and the cost far outweighed the modest saving.

Gender: Lastly, the principles allocate gender-specific roles. There is an explanation in the text, drawn from the world of computer science, but divorced from the principles. In a people-focused service such as healthcare, it is far more acceptable to use non-gender language.

The Final Analysis

The final analysis must be that the BMA addressed a major threat - an interactive health network linking electronic patient records - with the seriousness it deserved. However, rather than focusing on the immediate threat, it then addressed a deeper and wider issue of general confidentiality in electronically held records with undue haste and a technocratic view. The result lacks balanced underpinning by scientific analysis or patient opinion, could be prejudicial to effective care delivery, and would divert significant but unquantified resources (including clinician time) from direct care delivery in order to address an unquantified threat, without examining alternative approaches.

Ethically, the proposed principles are compromised. From a deontological viewpoint they are sound if, and only if, they have been thought through from every type of patient interest, which does not appear to be the case. From a utilitarian viewpoint they are seriously flawed, as they would reduce patient care volume by diverting resources with no proven gain, and would inhibit current good practice and quality assurance procedures. Again, this points to the problems of emergency value setting and policy making, and the iniquity of one body having to take on a societal and pan-professional role. This retrospective analysis should not be seen as petty problem-hunting, but rather as a salutory reminder of the complexity of health care services, the all-pervasive role of information, and consequently of the need for sound, practical yet effective, control compatible with the interests of individuals. It is a situation which other services, and other countries, will wish to avoid.

Restoring Confidence through Opportunity

However, the purpose of this paper is not to avoid the key issue - that of controlling the beneficial power of information technology in health so that it is not used malevolently, by accident or design. The medical profession has a key voice but not a monopoly, and for instance the occupational therapy profession in the U.K. has established a means of setting a lead for its members, and providing regular guidance, including discussion of computer confidentiality issues[28]. Above all, though, it is essential in a service about people to focus the debate and solutions upon the individual and their interests. Moreover, it is important that confidentiality is protected in a way which establishes public confidence, yet is clear to all, and enhances rather than impedes good care - namely by having clear and intelligible key principles. Additionally, this should not be seen as a reaction to control computer systems.

A security culture needs to pervade, but in a constructive way, seeing information technology as a protector more than as a threat. In the context of this case study, and recognising the sensitivity of personal health information, this is put forward in this final section in a health care context. However, this is seen as a potential generic approach, applicable similarly to other areas of sensitive personal information processing and storage.

A Patient Care Based Approach

A patient based approach is possible, and indeed an example of a working policy in the challenging setting of community care for citizens from birth to death has been put before the BMA's then Information Technology Working Party and found to be helpful[29]; this included a diagrammatic algorithm meaningful to public and staff, which also provided the logic for computer-based controls, protecting confidentiality whilst allowing carefully controlled staff supervision, with a degree of patient-based choice. In health care an effective approach needs to meet four key criteria: to be patient focused; to relate to good clinical processes; to exploit the power of computers to monitor and enforce security; and appropriate backing by legal and professional sanctions. Based on these criteria a practical model can be put forward based on true principles.

Confidentiality Protection Principles

The following nine Confidentiality Protection Principles are suggested for further open consideration. They seek to provide core values and objectives to underpin the development of a new paradigm for the new information technology, patient focused and clear to all parties.

1. Restriction to Involved Clinicians should be the prime principle of confidentiality:
A person's full health record should only be accessed by a health professional with a clinical need to know created by their having a duty-of-care for that person: such duty of care can only be created by patient presentation, by personal eligibility for a preventive health programme, by referral from a clinician already having a duty-of-care, or by shared team or locum responsibility linked to a clinician already involved (exceptions may be made as at present for pressing reasons of safety of a person, detection of serious crime, or national security, but these will be properly authorised and documented).
(Computer systems should only allow access on the basis or current involvement, including membership of a currently involved clinical team, or locum coverage for an involved clinician; as far as possible medical record librarians should operate similar policies for paper records.)

2. Acceptance of Personally Requested Special Levels of Confidentiality should be possible:
Though each person's health record should be confidential to the healthcare provider organisation (e.g. practice or trust), or to any smaller operational unit as defined in the confidentiality protection policy, and furthermore only accessed by those of its staff directly involved with the individual's care, patients may request that specific episodes or information items are even further restricted to a single health professional or team, but with counselling as to the possible adverse effects for the safety or effectiveness of future care.
(Protocols for hiding episodes, or for highly confidential notes, must be specified in the confidentiality protection policy.)

3. Restriction to Organisational Boundaries should be the basis of record control:
Personal health records created within one health care provider will be created for use only within that organisation, except for appropriate items being passed on as part of a referral, wherever possible with the subject's involvement. Subsequent requests by other external clinicians with a duty-of-care will be considered in the clinical interests of the patient, and any original patient request for enhanced confidentiality taken into account. External interrogation or other record access should not be permitted, except where authored messages for specific individuals are left for collection in a *poste restante* facility and released on authentication of identity.
(In the NHS the practice or Trust is the statutory body; team working involving staff of other agencies, and relationships with general practitioners particularly with regard to shared care, should be defined and published in the confidentiality protection policy.)

4. <u>Care Supervision and Development</u> should be part of the service provision:
Patients should be advised that supervision of staff and improving organisational performance are part of sound practice in ensuring delivery of good quality health care, and this may on occasions necessitate a health professional supervisor checking part of their record.
(The confidentiality protection policy should specify the controls exercised in supervisory and quality assurance procedures.)

5. <u>Operational Support Staff work within clear Parameters</u>:
Patients should be advised that clinicians need secretarial and similar support, and that financial claims for reimbursement of treatment costs also have to be made and verified, but that all staff involved in support have access only to the minimum necessary information, are supervised by a clinician, and are subject to severe sanctions should they misuse information.
(Each provider must have clear operational policies, including an effective confidentiality clause in all contracts of employment.)

6. <u>Audit Trails</u> should be part of the personal record:
All electronic record systems should have automated and tamper-proof audit trails which record all activity, including look-up access as well as creation and updating of records; these audit trails should be considered part of the individual record and therefore be available to the patient under statutory subject access provisions.
(This will provide legal right of access, but organisations will need to develop means of advising the benefits of focusing a search, and means of producing an intelligible printed version.)

7. <u>Physical Protection of Information</u> is part of information security: Patients should be advised of the measures to provide physical protection of their records from accidental or malicious loss or corruption; this should include fire and entry detection, and automated monitoring of computer activity.
(Risk analyses and countermeasures should be part of the technical specification of the confidentiality protection protocol.)

8. <u>Confidentiality Protection Policy Publication</u> is essential:
Each person wishing to receive services from a healthcare provider shall be able to obtain as a matter of course a copy of the organisation's confidentiality protection policy, written in consumer terms; this should be based on a technical specification, including computer system control protocols, and audit procedures.

(Each provider must have a formally ratified, technically specified policy, including system access control and verification procedures, differential data access controls, and automated monitoring of electronic record activity. A summary leaflet form should be displayed in access points, and included in appointments and admission packs.)

9. CONFIDENTIALITY POLICY PERFORMANCE should be published:
Each person shall be able to request a copy of the annual confidentiality protection audit report.
(Each provider should have an audit and monitoring procedure, including an annual report which should include summary of investigations, complaints, breaches of policy, and action taken.)

Harnessing The Computer's Contribution

The current debate is about stopping inappropriate use of information technology's potential power to harm confidentiality. However, computers can themselves also be harnessed to enhance both security and confidentiality in a way which is impossible with paper records. Space does not permit a full analysis of the issues and opportunities, but they can (and should) include:

- controlling who can access the record system
- controlling which types of information they can access
- controlling activity (ability to read, add to, or create)
- controlling who can access any individual record within the system
- enforcing tighter confidentiality when requested
- recording and attributing all activity, including reading as well as recording
- detecting unusual patterns of activity per terminal, staff member, or patient record
- enabling "back up" duplicate records to be maintained in a separate safe environment

Legal and Professional Sanctions

Good practice, and prevention of breach of confidentiality, are the optimum approaches. However, ability to fall back upon effective sanctions is an important part of the armoury. In the U.K. the Data Protection Act (1984) and the Computer Misuse Act (1990) are both invaluable, in that they make criminal offences the misuse of computer-held data, and seeking unauthorised access to electronic data, respectively. However, neither gives legal protection to patient confidentiality as a concept. This deficit would be addressed by the draft bill proposed by the BMA[30].

Professional bodies also provide a control over errant behaviour of health professionals, with the ultimate sanction of removing their right to practice if unprofessional activity is proven. Sanctions over support staff and others not operating under professional registration control are less satisfactory, pending appropriate legislation, but high store must be placed in contract of employment clauses and procedures, and indeed these have been used effectively, though this is not well known because of an understandable reluctance by all parties to seek publicity.

Generic Nature

These practice based principles are phrased in healthcare terms, as that this paper's setting, but they are generic in concept. By substituting other professional personnel and services in the text, they can be applied equally well, and favourably for the consumer, in any service or commercial setting. They are intended to be a means of focusing confidentiality on the consumer and their concerns, restricted to those directly involved, with the widening of the circle being on an identified 'when necessary' basis to specific persons for specific reasons.

Further Consideration

Clearly, further work on patient-based, computer-enhanced security is needed to develop universally clear and accepted principles and standards; the ideas put forward in this paper are offered as a foundation. Also, there must be mature discussion on issues such as service management, and the means of funding and controlling health care organisations - whether publicly or privately financed. These are issues where it is all too easy to say that patient confidentiality is absolute, without considering implications in terms of the interests of patients in having well-planned, responsive, and good quality health services.

However, though important, these topics are tangential to the primary concern - that of ensuring that patient record keeping is modern and effective, empowering and assisting the clinician by presenting the relevant information in a timely and accurate manner for the benefit of the patient, whilst also accommodating the patient's right to confidentiality in a context and manner they understand. These are functions which can be improved significantly by appropriate application of information technology.

Conclusion

As indicated in the first part of this paper, none of the parties involved with the current debate about the English NHS Information Management and Technology Strategy emerge with unimpeded vision. Positions have been clouded by extraneous factors including inappropriate haste. The patient has been referred to paternalistically, but neither consulted nor built in as the focus of the confidentiality model. Computers have been seen as solutions to unsought issues as well as to improving care, rather than as tools to be harnessed in a wider sense including policing their own activity. Scientific evidence and empirical analyses on benefits, and on drawbacks, have been lacking though appropriate techniques exist.

However, there is clear scope to move forward in a constructive way, with patient-based principles, strengthening good practice, and with much more informed and innovative harnessing of computers to provide confidentiality protection than has hitherto been possible with paper systems. Fundamental citizen-based principles can be framed and debated, and can provide the foundation for practical and enforcible rules.

From this case study can be learned lessons applicable far more widely than English healthcare, and principles emerge which are generic for the protection of personal information without jeopardising the effectiveness of the services citizens seek. Such a positive and responsible approach must be taken. Not to harness proven benefits of computing, or to make such use impractical or otherwise detrimental to patient care, is as unethical as to install unsafe applications.

References

1 Wilde O: Lady Windermere's Fan.

2 NHS Management Executive Information Management Group: An Information Management and Technology Strategy for the NHS in England - Getting Better with Information; Department of Health, Leeds, 1993.

3 Banta HD, Schersten T, Jonsson E: Implications of Minimally Invasive Therapy; Health Policy, 23, 167-178, 1993.

4 Anderson R: Clinical System Security: Interim Guidelines; British Medical, Journal, 312, 109-111 (1996).

5 NHS Management Executive: Computerisation in GP Practices 1993 Survey; Department of Health, Leeds, 1993.

6 M.J. Rigby: Decisions, Please (Item on strategic policy issues on information); The Health Summary, IX, II, 5-6, London, February 1992.

7 M. Rigby: NHS Information Handicap Stakes; The Health Summary, X, X, 4-6, October 1993.

8 Rigby M., Robins S: Community Health - Delivering the Vision; British Journal of Healthcare Computing and Information Management, 1994, 11, 6, 34-36.

9 Department of Health: Draft Guidelines on Confidentiality; Department of Health , London, 1994.

10 Department of Health: The Protection and Use of Patient Information: Department of Health, London, 1996.

11 Royal College of Psychiatrists: Report of the Mental Health Information Systems Working Group, Royal College of Psychiatrists, London, 1992.

12 Audit Commission: For Your Information - A Study of Information Management and Systems in the Acute Hospital; H.M.S.O., London, 1995.

13 Molteno B: Is Our Clinical Information Safe?; British Journal of Healthcare Computing and Information Management, 12, 12, 40-42.

14 Smith J: Personal Communications, 1995.

15 Anderson RJ: Security in Clinical Information Systems; British Medical Association, London, 1996

16 Personal communication, 1996.

17 Personal communication, 1996.

18 Institute of Medicine: The Computer-Based Patient Record - An Essential Technology for Health Care (Dick RS, Steen EB, eds.); National Academy Press, Washington DC, 1991.

19 Drazen EL et al: Patient Care Information Systems; Springer-Verlag, New York, 1995.

20 Bussey AL, Holmes B: Immunisation Levels and the Computer; Lancet, i, 450,1978.

21 Sullivan F, Mitchell E: Has General Practice Computing Made a Difference to Patient Care? - A Systematic Review of Published Reports; British Medical Journal, 311, 848-852, 1995.

22 Welsh Project Nurses Forum: Implementation of Nurse Information Systems - Benefits Assessment Studies, A Practical Guide; Welsh Health Common Services Authority, Cardiff, 1992.

23 Roger-France F, Noothoven van Goor J, Staer-Johansen K: Case-Based Telematic Systems Towards Equity in Health Care (Studies in Health Technology and Informatics Vol. 14); IOS Press, Amsterdam, 1994.

24 Rigby MJ, Robins SC: A Networked Patient-Based Integrated Care System as a Basis for the Achievement of Quality in Practice; in Roger-France F, Noothoven van Goor J, Staer-Johansen K: Case-Based Telematic Systems Towards Equity in Health Care (Studies in Health Technology and Informatics Vol. 14); IOS Press, Amsterdam, 1994.

25 Roberts R, Thomas J, Rigby M, Williams JG: Practical Protection of Confidentiality in Acute Healthcare; Paper to Cambridge University / BMA Conference on the Security of Personal Information, Cambridge University, Cambridge, 1996 (and reproduced in this volume).

26 Fowler HW, Fowler FG (eds.): The Concise Oxford Dictionary of Current English (Fifth edition); Oxford University Press, Oxford, 1964.

27 Maxwell RJ: Quality Assessment in Health; British Medical Journal, 288, 1470-1472, 1984.

28 Austin C: Confidentiality, Clinicians, and Computers; British Journal of Occupational Therapy, 59 (2), 62-64, 1996.

29 Rigby MJ: Electronic Patient records - Confidentiality, Access, and the 'Need to Know', a discussion paper; Plymouth Community Services NHS Trust, Plymouth, 1995.

30 British Medical Association: A Bill Governing Collection, Use and Disclosure of Personal Health Information; British Medical Association, London, 1995.

Electronic Patient Records : Usability vs Security, with Special Reference to Mental Health Records

Ronald J. Draper MA., MD., FRCPsych., FRCP(C)

Consultant Psychiatrist, St. John of God Order and Research Associate, Department of Psychiatry, University of Dublin. Formerly Professor of Psychiatry, University of Ottawa. and Clinical Birector, Brockville Psychiatric Hospital

1 Introduction

Medicine has entered a new era of fiscal restraint. The unspeakable is now reality and physicians must now temper their Hippocratic traditions with the realities of the market place where there are competing agendas. The funding agencies strive for efficiency, a commercial term implying doing more with less, and the providers strive to increase the effectiveness of their interventions through a process of continuous quality improvement. Both agendas require up to date clinical information to supports their arguments and achieve a best compromise division of the finite funding envelope. The complexity and sophistication of the data which will be required will be beyond the capacity of existing manual systems. Electronic data collection, storage, retrieval and processing will play an increasingly important role in clinical information systems and the new evidence based medicine.

The computer systems developed during the past decade were all successful in meeting statutory data requirements but were seen as 'business systems' by clinicians. Because of their administrative origins the clinical components were relatively poorly developed and largely failed to encourage clinicians to abandon their traditional practices, especially in fields such as mental health. This reluctance was justified for a variety of reasons; the text based screens were visually unattractive to the untrained eye, the architecture was often a computerised version of manual systems, because of uncertainty the two were often run in parallel adding to workload rather than relieving it, data was often not available on line. Finally the potential of the computer to do things differently was not properly exploited. The educational preparation required to change attitudes and practices was lacking. People were trained to use the new systems without first being introduced to the new electronic culture and shown how to exploit the new opportunities it offered.

Anyone who has ever had to retrieve data from conventional hand written patient records will be aware of the difficulties involved. Page follows page in a sequential, or linear, format. Pages are often poorly, even haphazardly, assembled and often illegible. Frequently the most important data are missing. No where is this problem more serious than in the mental health field where patients with long histories of multiple care episodes may have several volumes of records. Volume can correlate poorly with quality. There is a spurious notion of a comprehensive record. Virtually all data in manual files is in narrative format little changed since the days when wonderful prosaic descriptions were penned by those who first recognised diseases. Today such records are virtually useless for justifying and allocating budgets or supporting research. It is a sad fact too that in court many defenses of negligence claims fail because the clinical record has not documented key information. The problem is frequently on of omission rather than commission. Clearly the time is ripe for change and the electronic record is the putative agent for change. The author is currently employed in developing the specification for an Electronic Patient Record and Clinical Information System which will build on current experience and exploit future potential in a user friendly manner which will be described later. This paper will examine the various issues which impact Personal Information Security today.

2 Issues

2.1 Consent

During the first part of this century the focus of attention in respect of the mentally ill remained their care and management. This was still the age of the asylum. 1917 saw the introduction of a treatment for neurosyphilis followed by the introduction of electroconvulsive treatment in 1936 which was to prove an effective treatment for major depressive illness. Thus psychiatry began to emerge as a medical discipline. Further progress was however to wait until after the second world war. Following the revelations of wartime abuse of human rights and the subsequent Nuremberg trials of Nazi war criminals a doctrine of consent began to emerge and was refined and codified by the Declaration of Helsinki. The doctrine became more relevant to psychiatry with the introduction of psychoactive agents, antipsychotics and antidepressants, in the 1950's and 60's. The doctrine was stated very explicitly in the Canadian Charter of Rights and Freedoms which guarantees, inter alia, the right to life, liberty and freedom of the person. This right has been the basis for many challenges of detention, administration of drugs and ECT, disclosure of personal information. The resultant body of case law has fine tuned and clarified issues around consent which to be valid must be informed. The conflict between the new demands for transparent government and individual privacy resulted in a Freedom of Information and Protection of Privacy Act.

The issue is that there is no absolute guarantee of either right but a compromise between them.

2.2 Competence

All legislation addresses individuals presumed to be competent to understand, appreciate and utilise the concepts involved. The corollary is the assumption that if people do so understand and avail of the various protections, the law has achieved it's purpose. In mental illness this assumption may be very unwise. Psychiatry deals with severely ill patients, those whose thought processes have been disturbed by mental illness or organic impairment, who may be quite unable to understand or correctly interpret information. The legislation does not speak to them. There can be no informed consent. In many jurisdictions Mental Health Acts require formal tests of competence, or capacity, to consent. A practical schema was developed by Draper & Dawson (199) which comprises a decision tree based upon:

2.3 Providing information

- Testing the patient's insight as to whether the are mentally ill.
- Ascertaining whether they understand the benefits of the proposed treatment,
- Ascertaining whether they understand the consequences of not accepting,
- Ascertaining their ability to maintain a fixed choice.

If the patient is found not competent a substitute consenter must be found from a hierarchy laid down in the Mental Health Act and this person must act according to a specified 'best interests' process.

The issue is that access controls must allow for non competent patients and the involvement of substitute consenters and second opinions.

2.4 The Medical Record

When the Joint Commission for the Accreditation of Hospitals in the US and it's sister organisation, the Canadian Council for Hospital Accreditation began work a quarter of a century ago a principle focus was the quality of medical records. Standards were developed and random audits continue to this day. The standards have evolved and have been expanded but essentially define the purposes of a medical record as:

- To accurately identify the patient,
- To acquire and record all information necessary to establish a comprehensive diagnosis and treatment plan,
- To record all actions undertaken for, by, or on behalf, of the patient,
- To provide a means of accurate communication between all professionals involved in the patient's care and treatment,
- To provide a continuous record of the patient's treatment, investigations and progress,

  To these should now be added
- To highlight behavioral and physical 'alerts',
- To support a continuous quality improvement process.

To this day professional Licensing and Certification bodies remain concerned about the quality of medical records and deficient records remain a major source of malpractice claims. Courts find themselves in great difficulty when they are assured by defendants that such and such took place in a particular way yet there is no record of the event. A recent high profile action in the Republic of Ireland was successful for this very reason.

The issue is the necessity for access controls to accommodate the structure and function of a medical record, which must be able to generate both cross sectional and longitudinal data.

Any attempt to exclude portions of the record could have disastrous consequences if say, homicidal/suicidal behaviour, life threatening drug reactions etc., were hidden from the treating professionals. This argues the absolute necessity for records to be:

- comprehensive,
- continuous - especially if the patient receives care in a variety of settings and locations.

2.5 The nature of Practice

The traditional view of medicine is of a single decision maker, the doctor, who is assisted by nurses and others who carry out his/her instructions. Mental health is one discipline which has departed radically from this concept. By the middle of this century mental health acts had changed to allow voluntary treatment. Alternatives to hospital began to develop. The age of community psychiatry was dawning. The new drugs were successful in controlling major mental illness. Optimism was the order of the day. Patients began to be discharged into the community. After the debacle of deinstitutionalisation in the 1950's and 60's it was realised that merely controlling psychotic symptoms was not enough. Patients had to be prepared for life in the community and the community had to be educated and resourced to allow them to rejoin society. Their needs were now recognised to be multiple. The focus began to shift from a medical model to a biopsychosocial one in which many disciplines and skills were required. The multidisciplinary team evolved. Decision making was now dispersed albeit coordinated. This was the basis for the Assertive Community Team developed by Stein and Test in Wisconsin US, replicated by Hoult and Reynolds in New South Wales and Burti et al in S. Verona. The approach has been highly successful in reducing the need for hospital care by providing to patients the services they need, where they need them, when they need them. Typically providing service around the clock. Such teams have been shown to score as well as or better that hospital based programs on measures of Patient Satisfaction and Quality of Life. The approach is now widely disseminated and will be a major feature of future mental health services. This success depends heavily upon a multidisciplinary team being able to readily access, communicate and share patient information.

The issue is that access controls must provide for care being provided by groups of professionals rather than individual decision makers.

2.6 Quality

The accreditation process in North America has driven a quality improvement agenda. Today no hospital or health care facility can be accredited without having a well developed quality assurance program which meets strict explicit standards. Governments have supported this development, often enthusiastically, one suspects that for them their ability to demonstrate a commitment to quality is a useful mask for their plundering of mental health budgets in the name of efficiency. In the UK and Ireland patient charters have been developed. Acronyms abound in this field. The seminal Quality Control QC is an industrial concept, at it's simplest ensuring that, for example, all the nuts and bolts in a packet match. The next step was Quality Assurance QA , ensuring that something did or did not happen. This was the start of medical quality assurance. Initially it was structural e.g.., checking to see that the fire extinguishers had been checked or that all of the correct solutions were in the radiology department. Next it was process, looking at how thing worked whether in the laboratory or on the ward. Neither activity correlated with quality care. Finally came the realisation that it was necessary to measure outcomes if one was to really measure quality of care. In order to do so it is first necessary to develop indicators against which outcomes can be measured. This has been done extensively in physical and laboratory medicine. Mental health has presented an entirely different challenge which has deterred most. Because of the multidisciplinary nature of practice coupled with many and varied goals the search for valid indicators has been arduous. Finally a methodology has emerged - the Strategic Planning Approach. This is an ongoing, constantly updating process which starts with a needs assessment (of community needs or individual needs). This informs the Mission Statement which is a statement of services to be provided and to whom. Next come the organisation's goals or aspirations which give rise to time limited, measurable objectives. Activities or programs are tailored to meet the objectives. The outcomes are then measured against the original objectives and evaluated. The evaluation results then feedback to inform and if necessary revise, the Mission Statement. This is a circular and continuous process which is also the basis of care planning

2.7 Strategic planing

The Strategic plan is an integral part of Continuous quality improvement (synonym: Total quality management) which has a series of component parts:

Quality Assurance (QA) : patient outcome evaluation; program outcome evaluation

Quality Management (QM) : developing strategic and operational plans, which produce quality outcomes for the patients which the organisation serves

Utilisation Management (UM) : maximising the effectiveness and efficiency with which the organisation's resources are allocated

Risk Management (RM): minimising liability and loss through preventive identification and control of risks.

The key to these processes is information. Coding, standardisation and numeration of clinical information is essential. There is a trade off between access to patient records and improved quality of care.

2.8 Economics

A study by the World Bank and the World Health Organisation published in 1993 concluded that the total burden of mental disorders is greater than that caused by cancer. Approximately 10 which means that at any one time 450 million people suffer from a severe neuropsychiatric problem. There is every reason to believe that mental health problems will grow faster than populations in both developed and under developed countries (Gulbinat, 1994). Three 'entry points' are identified for increasing the cost effectiveness of health care:

- to optimise at treatment level the interplay between problem assessment, intervention and outcome
- at Regional / National level to optimise the organisation of health care
- to invest in research in order to find better ways of organising health care provision

The basis for all of these processes is information. Gulbinat (1994) identifies 4 types of computer based mental health information systems:

- Stand alone workstation
- Limited network of work stations (e.g.. a hospital)
- Hospital wide electronic record system
- Regional or National electronic patient record system.

The Audit Commission found that medical and nursing staff in acute care settings spend up to 25collecting, analysing, using, and communicating information. Mental health staff may well spend an even greater proportion of their time so engaged. Despite this enormous resource allocation records remain dispersed, poorly integrated, incomplete and lacking standardisation. Clinical audit invariably finds that important clinical items are incomplete or missing altogether (Lelliott, 1995). The potential to use computers to improve completeness and accuracy, free up time, and develop true personal health care records, which would minimise duplication and enhance quality of care is enormous and as yet poorly exploited.

The issue is that increasing cost effectiveness requires computer based systems.

2.9 Research

Computers are now recognised to be essential tools in research but many clinicians do not appreciate their role in the clinical setting. It is suggested , however, that in medicine clinical and research activities should not be greatly distinguished, especially in psychiatry, because so much remains unknown. Treatment response rates in most diagnoses rarely exceed 60 - 70

The issue is that 'the successful integration of research methods with clinical practice lies in the use of computers'.

2.10 Evidence based care

Computers are poised to become key players in the delivery of health care. They have the potential to assist in diagnosis, provide continuous medical education, disseminate evidence and research findings, simplify practice management, and make it more efficient. Computers will be a cornerstone of evidence based care, touted as the medicine of the future. Physicians will be aware of all evidence available to support therapeutic decisions and evaluate them. Practice will move from heavy reliance upon intuition to use evidence from controlled trials and from the histories physicians take from their patients and the observations they make when examining them (Lowry, 1995). It is all about integrating individual clinical experience with the best external evidence. British centres for Evidence based practice have been established or planned in a number of specialties (Sackett et al, 1996).

Best practice will be dependent upon the use of computers.

3 Imperatives

All of the afore going processes, Consent, Competence, The Medical Record, The Nature of Practice, Quality improvement, Economics, Research, Evidence based learning, argue for broad access to the clinical record which is essential for their effective functioning. There are obviously other arguments in favour of restricting or denying access in the interests of security and confidentiality.

3.1 Security

Security of electronic media has been a concern from the start when the American Military set up ARPAnet. The concern was that a central hub would be vulnerable to destruction. The solution chosen was a network of computers which would allow data to be re-routed if one or two units were destroyed. Gradually the net expanded to embrace many other government institutions Other networks were being developed in the early 1980's and the ' network of networks' was named the Internet (Littlejohns & Briscoe 1996). Subsequent growth was phenomenal. From 300 hosts and 250 networks detected in 1981 to 3,000.000 hosts and 50,000 networks in 1994 (Cheswick & Bellovin 1994). Unlawful attempts to penetrate network security , hacking, were initially focused upon military secrets but as the I-net expanded commercial and finally personal secrets became vulnerable. Some attempts, because of their high profile nature raised fears for the security of electronic information which must be allayed if people are to be comfortable with electronic storage of their personal information.

Amorosa (1994) has provided an attack taxonomy:

- External Information Theft (glancing at someone's terminal)
- External Abuse of Resources (physical damage to the system)
- Masquerading (recording and playing back network transmissions)
- Pest Programs (installing a malicious program)
- Bypassing Authentication or Authority (password cracking)
- Authority Abuse (falsifying records)
- Abuse Through Inaction (intentionally bad management)
- Indirect Abuse (using another system to create a malicious program)

He believes that three factors have to be considered in considering system security.

- Threats
- Vulnerabilities
- Attacks

. He defines a threat as "any potential occurrence, malicious or otherwise, that can have an undesirable effect on the assets and resources associated with a computer system".

A vulnerability of a computer system is " some unfortunate characteristic that makes it possible for a threat to occur" thus threats can be mitigated by identifying and removing vulnerabilities.

An attack on a computer system is " some action taken by a malicious intruder that involves the exploitation of certain vulnerabilities in order to cause an existing threat to occur".

Threats can be classified into several categories:

- Disclosure (leak)
- Integrity (unauthorised changes to system or information)
- Denial of service (blocking of authorised use).

Common attack methods include:

- Password spoof programs
- Password theft by clever reasoning
- Logic bomb mail
- Scheduled file removal
- Field separator attack
- Insertion of compiler Trojan Horse

Another way of classifying security failures is to group them into two classes:

- Accidental
- Intentional

Accidental events include, Errors and Omissions, power failures, cable cuts, fire, flood, earth movement, solar flares, volcanoes, severe weather, static electricity, lightning, relocation, maintenance, testing, humidity, smoke, dust, gasses, fumes, cleaning chemicals, heat, temperature cycling, electronic interference, vibration, corrosion. A long list of intentional events is also detailed (Cohen, 1995). Cohen's list of accidental events is useful because it illustrates the point that system security deals with more than electronic threats. It has been estimated (Cohen, 1995) that the FBI calculation of $ 5 billion annual loss to computer crime is but the tip of the iceberg. This need not be if available security techniques are employed. Excellent texts are available on System Security Engineering (Amorosa, 1994), Integrity Mechanisms (Cohen, 1995), "Firewall' gateways (Cheswick & Bellovin 1994), Protecting and rebuilding Networks (Held, 1995). Cheswick & Bellovin paraphrase Grampp & Morris "It is easy to run a secure computer system. You merely have to disconnect all dial up connections and permit only hard wired terminals, put the machine and it's terminals in a shielded room, and post a guard at the door". The point is simple - there is no such thing as a 100

There is an inevitable trade-off between security and usability. That is, a conflict generally occurs when the goal of information and resource sharing is combined with the goal of strict security between users (Amorosa, 1994)". We must not , however, allow the wonders of technology to blind us to some basic facts about human behaviour. Not all attacks, perhaps only a small minority, are launched via electronic media. One that led to the termination of a US presidency involved theft of manual records. Reports of the routine sale of personal health information for as little as =9C 150 have been noted (Anderson , 1996). Even if a computer has no electronic links it is not necessarily secure. Simple attack prevention methods (Amorosa ,1994) include:

Individual Screening This method involves checking the background, credentials, family and other personal attributes of all individuals who can attack a system. The goal is to only grant access to those who can be trusted.

Physical Controls These involve securing the facility and surroundings of a computer system.

Care in Operations Failure to protect passwords, failure to clear screens before log in, leaving files open, leaving terminals unattended, lack of education/training in security, poorly designed access controls, lax administration are all threats. Carelessness about telephone enquiries is one of the main threats to general practice systems (Anderson 1996).

All of these strategies have their counterparts in the security of manual records.

The issue is not whether electronic records can be perfectly secure but rather whether computer systems can be designed to provide better security that manual records.

Having been concerned with the protection of electronic records the European Commission (1995) now makes no distinction between the "processing of personal data wholly or partly by automatic means, and to the processing otherwise than by automatic means which form part of a filing system or are intended to form part of a filing system (Article 3 (1))". The status quo is simply no longer an option.

Lelliott (1995) has summarised the advantages of computer systems and the Key Principles of the Information Management and Technology Strategy (IMG, 1992) which are that:

- There will be a health care record for every person who has a NHS number.
- Data will be entered only once and shared with other NHS designated systems.
- Information will be captured from health care professional's daily work.
- Information will be secure and confidential.
- Common standards and NHS-wide networking will allow computers to share information.

This concept of a NHS-wide network seems to have brought the NHS Executive's information management group into conflict with the ethical position of the BMA and the guidance from the joint computer group of the BMA and the Royal College of General Practitioners. The development of extensive systems in Mental Health will pose further problems and involve the Royal College of Psychiatrists. The guidelines involve nine principles of data security. It may be possible to operationalise them on general practice systems for which they are clearly designed but any attempt to generalise them to other fields, particularly Mental Health could be disastrous and tip the balance of usability vs protection to an unacceptable extent. The functioning of multidisciplinary teams would be greatly obstructed if not vitiated. There is going to have to be dialogue too in relation to the Data Protection Acts (UK, 1984), (Ireland, 1988) and regulations attached thereto.

4 St. John of God

The Hospitaller Order of St. John of God operates a major psychiatric hospital at Stillorgan Co. Dublin which admits both private and public patients on an equal basis. It operates the catchment area psychiatric service to 161,000 residents of Dublin South East on behalf of the Eastern Health Board and a wide area Child Psychiatry service based in South Dublin. These facilities are all several miles apart and operate on multiple sites with day facilities closing down after office hours. The Order decided that all of these services should be integrated into one mental health service. A major ongoing problem centered upon the availability of patient records. These tended to be located where the patient last attended and to be unavailable if the patient presented for after hours assessment/admission to hospital. The development of the specification for an electronic patient record EPR and clinical information system CIS is now well advanced. Lelliott at al

(1993) reviewed seven leading mental health information systems on behalf of the Royal College of Psychiatrists. Neither these nor several newer developments will support the St. John of God specification in their present forms.

4.1 Specification

The specification is considered to be innovative. It is comprehensive and currently encompasses all aspects of mental health in both hospital and community settings. It attempts to utilise the computer to build added value into all areas of operation for example, one objective is to have a quantitative record. The system will have both LAN and WAN networks but with available security methodology and encryption techniques system security is seen as a challenge which can be met.

Development currently has three strands:

- The specification
- Development of access controls and audit trails
- Legal, ethical, and data protection.

The specification has been developed using a bottom up approach to person based records which share the key principles of the Information Management & Technology Strategy (Lelliott, 1995). An interactive consultation process has been developed using large and small groups in planning cycles to involve staff in the development of their system.

Access to the system by authorised user names and personal ID codes will be on a need to know basis with multiple levels of access appropriate to staff functions. Entries will be written on a read only basis, will have digital signatures, and generate audit trails. Data security and confidentiality will be a priority.

A legal, ethical, and data protection task force has been struck. The Irish Data Protection Act (1988) and regulations have a series of 8 provisions relating to the obtaining, purpose, safe keeping, use and disclosure, safety and security, accuracy and currency, adequacy and relevancy, retention, and right of access. In the UK Anderson (1996) has drawn up interim guidelines for the BMA. These include nine principles of data security. Of these 1 - 4 deal with access control, record opening, control and consent. These are likely to be controversial because of their restrictiveness which may be appropriate in general practice but would be impossible to operationalise in mental health. We believe that data protection is a different issue to system security and is primarily an issue of consent. The interim guidelines take a mechanistic approach which reduces consent to four steps which are locked rigidly into the security system. This approach does not address the quality of consent, whether it is informed or mere passive compliance. Neither does it address the issue of the non-competent patient. The alternative approach being adopted is to see data protection as an ethical and consent issue and develop mechanisms to inform patients and obtain their consent in a manner analogous to the schema described (Draper & Dawson, 1990) for testing competence.

5 Summary & Conclusions

The development of computerised patient records is being driven by a number of imperatives which have been identified. The growth of computer systems in health care will increase in pace and scope. Threats and attacks launched via electronic media have resulted in the development of effective mechanisms and strategies which allow systems to be designed with high levels of security

Computers are essential to support research and effective resource allocation in the interests of better patient care. Specifications can be developed to meet these goals. The development of an electronic patient record system will confront legal issues of admissibility as evidence, which are being addressed, and ethical issues of consent. There are competing agendas. Solutions will represent a trade off between usability and security. This is a reality which should be explicit and part of the patient information underpinning informed consent which includes explanation as to why data is being collected and the extensive measures taken to protect it. Mandatory consent will raise other legal issues such as the ability and wisdom of treatment on the basis of incomplete information.
Dublin 8 May 1996

6 References

Anderson Ross. Clinical system security: interim guidelines. BMJ 1996; 312: 109-111

Amoroso Edward. Fundamentals of computer security technology. Prentice-Hall: New Jersey, 1944

Cheswick W. R., Bellovin S. M. Firewalls and internet security. Addison-Wesley: New York, 1994

Cohen Frederick. Protection and security on the information superhighway. John Wiley & Sons: New York, 1995

Data Protection Act, Govt. of Ireland, 1988

Draper R., Dawson D. Competence to consent to treatment: guidelines for the psychiatrist. Canadian Journal of Psychiatry, 1990; 35(4): 285 - 289

European Commission, Directive 95/46/EC, 24 Oct. 1995

Gulbinat W. International standards in behavioral Informatics: issues and controversies. Computers in mental health. 1994, 1; 30 - 35

Held Gilbert. Protecting LAN resources. John Wiley & Sons: New York, 1995

Lelliott Paul. Mental health information systems: problems and opportunities. Advances in Psychiatric Treatment 1995; 1:216-222

Lelliott P., Flannigan C., Shanks S. A review of seven mental health information systems. Research Unit Publications (RUP 1). Royal College of Psychiatrists: London, 1993

Littlejohns C., Briscoe M. The information superhighway. Psychiatric Bulletin 1996; 20: 146-148

Lowry Fran. Computers a cornerstone of evidence-based care, conference told. Can. Med Assoc J. 1995, 153; 11: 1636-39

Sackett D. L., Rosenberg W. M. C., Muir Gray J. A., Haynes R. B., Richardson W. S. Evidence based medicine: what it is and what it isn't. BMJ.1996, 312; 71-72

Tien A. Y. Computers, communication and collaboration. Computers in Mental Health. 1994, 1; 24 - 29

Security and Confidentiality Issues Relating to the Electronic Data Interchange of Clinical Data

Peter Landrock,
Aarhus University & Newton Institute, Cambridge University

John Williams, GP, Guildford
Senior User to the GP/Provider Links Project

1. Introduction

The purpose of Electronic Data Interchange (EDI) is to communicate and process structured data in an automated fashion. General Practitioners (GPs) are overwhelmed with paper despite the fact that well over 80% have computerised clinical systems. Much of this paper derives from hospitals and other provider units. Some of it is carried on forms that could easily be replaced with EDI.

The GP/Provider Links Project (GPPL), which is part of the Patients Not Paper (PNP) initiative is charged with implementing the first three standard clinical EDIFACT messages that have so far received professional acceptance. PNP dictates that it should deliver implementation by December 31, 1996. The three EDIFACT messages in question are as follows:

1. Pathology requests and results
2. Radiology requests and results
3. Hospital referrals / discharges

In the first case GPs request laboratory tests such as full blood count, or liver function tests, or microscopy and culture of urine. Currently the appropriate specimen is taken from the patient, labelled, and sent with a hand completed request form (often by courier) to the laboratory. After running the relevant assay the laboratory then sends back the result either by post or by courier. Urgent results are often delivered over the telephone. Request forms typically carry the patients name, date of birth, and sometimes address. Depending on circumstances clinical information such as relevant current condition, past history and drug therapy may also be included. The chief advantage of EDI in this case is not so much faster turnaround but more the fact that requests and results can be handled by a paperless system with results more reliably matched to requests and patients. The results can then be automatically filed in a structured manner linked to the appropriate patients record. They are then readily accessible at subsequent consultations, and to decision support systems, and to structured reporting systems.

In the second case GPs request Xrays such as knee / wrist / abdomen of their local hospital Xray department. Currently request forms are filled in by hand with information very similar to that placed on pathology request forms. The request forms are typically conveyed to the hospital either by the patient, by post or by courier. The main benefits from an EDI solution would again be the elimination of paper, more reliable match of result to request, and report held in the GP clinical system in an easily accessible and appropriate part of the patients record.

In the third case GPs currently refer patients to their hospital colleagues. Usually a referral letter is dictated and then later typed on a word processor, sometimes linked to the relevant patients record. This will typically contain even more detailed personal information than either of the previous requests, including detailed clinical information covering almost any aspect of the patients current or past medical history. It is then sent by post or by courier to the hospital. In the hospital a wide variety of non clinical staff may handle this letter for administrative and contractual reasons. Subsequently a variety of clinical letters (including hospital discharge) may be generated by the consultant or by junior staff - more or less taking the reverse route of the referral letter. Advantages of automation would include reduction of paperwork, structured filing of outpatient and discharge letters in the patients electronic record making retrieval easier, and possibly faster notification of treatment on discharge.

In none of these cases will the proposed EDI solution be conveying any information that is not already exchanged on paper, and in every case there are benefits to patient care in terms of information being more readily accessible and the right information being more reliably attached to the right patients record.

2. Threats

As much other electronic communication, such EDI messages are typically communicated via different networks, public as well as private, which raises a number of security issues. There are some very strong ethical reasons why clinicians feel that clinical information should be protected against various threats, the most obvious being unintended disclosure of private information, which in fact would violate the new strict laws on privacy in Europe. Here the most obvious threat is most likely provided by the LANs if not properly protected rather than public networks, where timing is much more of an issue for successful eavesdropping on particular data.

Given that it is very realistic to be more concerned about snooping using promiscuous mode on various unprotected LANs than about the vulnerability in the public networks as a whole, there would need to be a clinical system capable of making sense of end-to-end encryption/decryption of EDIFACT messages. In other words, we need a robust solution that takes care of LANs as well as the WANs.

Independently of this each clinician needs to maintain responsibility for the security of the data once it leaves his/her domain. It should remain thus until it reaches its intended recipient. There is a need to authenticate messages as well and ensure that they have not been altered in transit or perhaps even be planted with malicious intention. Initially just pathology results, radiology results and hospital discharges will be implemented, but this may be extended later to include more critical data. For further discussion of the possible threats and remedies against these, we refer the reader to the BMA security policy ([1]).

At least for the time being, it seems reasonable to assume that a single General Practice may be considered a secure domain. In particular, in so far as confidentiality is concerned, it would make sense to have data which is received in encrypted form, decrypted in an automated fashion upon arrival at the GP server. Using public key techniques, this would imply that the public key of the GP site is distributed to the communication partners, and the corresponding private key for decryption is permanently installed on the GP server. This need not create any breach of confidentiality, as information on patients is stored in the clear anyway. Most people working at the GP site are entitled to read the information anyway.

The biggest problems seem to arise at the hospital end. One possibility likely to be considered by many NHS Trusts is to install one single X400 link - and to have an EDIFACT translator associated with it. This would lead to all messages being decrypted in one place immediately on receipt by X400 - so that they could all go to a single EDIFACT translator. But this would then mean distributing clinical information in the clear across what ever LAN system the NHS Trust might have and presumably losing the certainty of the authentication too. Since very large numbers of different people have access to such a LAN for a wide variety of different purposes, controlling who has access to what is likely to be very difficult.

Moreover, it is a problem to consider, that VAN-service providers may process a message - or translate it from one format to another, which is unacceptable when security features are added.

The alternative would be to devise some means of having clinical information disseminated across the Trust's LAN while still encrypted - which in turn implies the need for a distributed system of decryption software and EDIFACT translators. This is what is being proposed in this paper

In other applications, such as the recently completed worldwide pilot on electronic bills of lading, BOLERO, there is a similar requirement and interest in adding security at the EDIFACT level. Here the various users cannot even be assumed to have the same X.400 mail system, which means that security features simply cannot be implemented at this layer.

3. Security measures

3.1 Security services

Just as in the paper world, a number of security services, reflecting the requirements of the users, can been identified in electronic communication. The list is not static, and more and more services are identified, as the technology and known techniques improve. The standard source is ISO International Standard 7498-2: Open Systems Interconnection Reference Model - Part 2: Security Architecture, 1989.

Appending a hand-written signature to a document, mailing a registered letter, etc. are corresponding examples of applications of security services which are essential in the paper world.

The following services are relevant for EDI: (Definitions copied in part from ISO 7498-2 and "Recommendations for UN/EDIFACT message level security")

data integrity: The property that data has not been altered or destroyed in an unauthorized manner.

data, or message (origin) authentication: The corroboration that the source of data received is as claimed.

(peer) entity authentication: The corroboration that a peer entity in an association is the one claimed.

non-repudiation services: Prevents denial by one of the entities involved in a communication of having participated in all or part of the communication.

confidentiality: The property that information is not made available to disclosed to unauthorized individuals, entities, or processes.

The point of these services is of course that they reflect the user's needs, regardless - in principle - of whether he uses paper or EDI to communicate information.

A service, which is not directly relevant in EDI, is

3.2 Access control

Access control gives a user access to certain rights. This is typically the situation with magnetic credit cards. Indeed, when a credit card is used, there is not provable connection between the user and the data, only a presumed, or indicated connection, which in fact would not be detected, even if the data was replaced, unless the POS-terminal where the card is used, offers additional protection, such as cryptography (see below).

Of course, access control may be relevant in connection with supporting services in EDI, such as storage of EDI-messages.

It is a common misconception that access control methods such as PIN-codes and biometrics recognition provide some degree of message authentication. Access control provides an identification of an entity, but does not in itself establish a connection between an entity and electronic data. More is needed.

1. Pincodes or passwords are examples of access control or identification mechanisms. It may for instance give a person access to information on a chipcard (or smartcard) or a computer. However, if in fact they are used to encrypt an electronic document or create a fingerprint of a document, they provide authentication, but not a digital signature.

2. Biometrics can only provide identification (of an entity) and never authentication of electronic data. There is no connecting element, such as a key (see below)!

In conclusion, any kind of security service in EDI has to involve some tied connection between the entity and the data, which requires the use of cryptographic techniques. There is no other way. Access control mechanisms, such as PIN-codes, biometrics identification etc. can not provide this. They may be part of the whole procedure: A PIN-code may give access to a chipcard which contains the secret key by which a digital signature may be created.

3.3 EDIFACT Security

Recently, UN/EDIFACT has provided the first drafts of international standards (ISO 9735) for the integration of security into EDIFACT messages, be it integrity, message authentication, non-repudiation of origin/receipt of a message or confidentiality. Likewise a new message, KEYMAN, has been developed to handle key management messages within the EDIFACT environment. The big advantage is that not only the message content, but the security of the message content, whichever nature, can be handled at the spot where messages are being read or produced by authorised personnel. This approach is very much in line with the BMA security policy ([1]).

In the following, we will discuss the possible short, medium, and long term solutions in the above mentioned approach. The short term should allow the implementation to go forward in the interests of better patient care while the medium term might be to pilot more durable solution(s), one or more of which might become long term solutions.

It should be added, that at the time of publishing, NHS is conducting a pilot of this approach between selected GPs and Hospital Units.

4. The Technical Solution for Security

The idea of the approach is the following. Once the messages are generated by the application by the EDIFACT translator, based on the data supplied by the clinician or GP or whoever, in the following called the user for simplicity, the user can specify which messages in which interchanges should be protected by which security service.

At the transmitting end, this is the only visible part of the security. The actual cryptographic mechanism is then calculated by a special security front-end, as described below.

At the receiving end, the inverse mechanism or verification mechanism, depending on which security services has been applied is performed automatically by this front-end, provided the user has demonstration authority to access the data.

The SF management is responsible for intercepting incoming and outgoing messages and to determine how to process them based on input from the security application. Examples of such processing are: apply integrated security, add separate security, generate AUTACK (a special EDIFACT message to carry a digital signature) for non-repudiation of receipt, fetch certificate, verify signature etc. The processing is then performed by the EDIFACT security module (for secured messages), or the KEYMAN module or the X.500 interface module for key management messages if required.

The EDIFACT security module is used to generate/verify EDIFACT security messages (AUTACK's and/or interchanges with integrated security), and the X.500 interface module is used to fetch certificates from the X.500 directory.

Architecture based on the Security Front-end approach

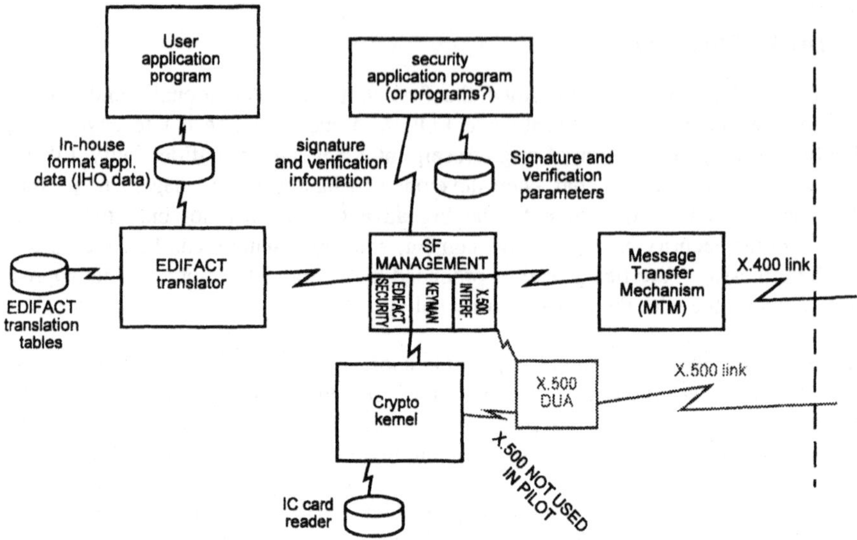

The crypto kernel is used to hash messages down, and (when chipcards are not used) sign or verify signatures. When chipcards are used, the signature generation and verification takes place on the card. The security submodule thus contains all the necessary cryptographic functions

4.1 Secure front-end

Apart from processing EDIFACT interchanges by means of the EDIFACT secure front-end, an interface must be available to the DUA (Directory User Agent), responsible for the communication set-up with the Directory, as well in the ultimate solution. This DUA will use the crypto kernel as a back-end, too. Furthermore it will be necessary to develop management procedures for the communication between these front-ends: it will be necessary to define how and when to use integrated certificates or locally stored certificates (in a cache or a database) or when to fetch certificates from directory and/or CA. However, in pilots, users will not need to access the Directory in a secure manner.

Information such as when to use which certificate could be stored along with the above mentioned information in the "security attribute and policy" database. The front-end can only verify that with a particular certificate, the verification of the signature is positive. It cannot decide if the certificate is the right one for a particular message.

4.2 Front-end security translator

4.2.1 Scope

A "Front-end Security Translator" to the EDIFACT-translators will handle security. This requires that an EDIFACT interchange can be intercepted after it has left the translator but before it is forwarded by X.400.

4.2.2 Purpose

The advantage of this solution is at least twofold:

a) The EDIFACT translators are used without integration of the security features, independently of which translator is used.

b) The EDIFACT security functions have been implemented as a completely separated module in ANSI-C and then integrated on any platform. In particular, the user platform application program will not communicate directly with the crypto-kernel.

4.2.3 Requirements and assumptions.

The requirements for taking the path with the security front end are the following.

1. It should be possible to intercept messages, i.e. the application should not be a CFA (Continuous Flow Application) type.
2. Interchanges are flagged by the front-end to indicate if security has been added.
3. An interchange, which contains messages to be secured must not be submitted by the translator until the security front-end has received the interchange reference number.
4. The front-end must be integrated in the system in such a way that it checks all interchange reference numbers.

5. Technical Specification of Security

Input/output EDIFACT front-end specification

5.1 At the transmitting end:

5.1.1 Input:

From user/user application:

Interchange reference number for interchange to be secured

Indication of whether non-repudiation of receipt is required

PIN-code to initiate the generation of a signature using the private key

From translator:

All interchanges.

5.1.2 Process and output:

- The Interchange is intercepted. Whenever an interchange passes, the front-end verifies if this interchange, as identified by the user application input, should be picked up for further security processing. (Alternatively, it might be safer that for all interchanges (or messages of certain types) the front-end inquires at the user which of the options (encryption / no encryption, signature/no signature) should be chosen.)

- If security has been required, input is forwarded to the EDIFACT SECURITY module for further processing, and a signature input is calculated by the crypto kernel, which is then forwarded for encryption. The secret keys could be secured on chipcards.
- If the PIN-code has been made available, a signature is calculated by the chipcard and returned, and then encrypted for confidentiality.
- If the signature is not returned within a certain period, specified as a parameter, the SF MANAGEMENT stores the interchange reference number and the chipcard input in an "Not signed" queue and proceed. If this happens the event is logged. This queue can always be reviewed, but this would require a call from the security application program.
- The last security service to be applied is encryption, if confidentiality is required.

5.2 At the receiving end:

5.2.1 Process and output:

- The first step is decryption, if confidentiality has been required. This will be handed in an automated fashion at the receiving work station, as explained earlier.
- If signed, the signature verification takes place. This involves verification of the certificate if included, as well as the signature. Alternatively, the public key needed for verification may have been exchanged on a bilateral basis. Otherwise, the received message will be stored in the appropriate stack.
- If the signature verification is successful, notification is forwarded to the user to inform which interchange was verified, and which certificate reference number was used, as well as the result of the verification, together with a query for further instruction. If the verification is unsuccessful, the nature of the failure is explained: Certification verification failed, signature failed.
- Furthermore, if non-repudiation of receipt is required, an AUTACK for acknowledgement is produced and returned to the transmitter.
- If an enclosed certificate is considered too old or otherwise requires further investigation, the interchange is put in a "wait" stack, and a query is forwarded to the Directory for the latest update on the status of the certificate For interchanges in the "wait" stack, the verification process is resumed, once this information is returned

6. Conclusion

We have explained how the fundamental requirement for privacy of patient related information requires that security is added as a genuine end-to end service, and that the solutions for this are there already.

It is a dramatic step to move away from paper based journals and information to electronic versions, as the protection of this information is so fragile unless profound precautions are taken. The primary goal to improve patient care cannot be over-emphasised. First and foremost we want working systems that enhance patient care, and secondly we want for the security and confidentiality features not to obstruct this primary aim.

Having stressed this, it is clear that adequate security features must be added, and this in a manner that data be equally well protected by cryptographic means -the only means - in LANs as in WANs. This means integration of security services as part of the EDIFACT-application, and the solutions are there, they have been chosen for the same reasons in a number of commercial projects, the standards are in place, and the cost could - and indeed should - be minimal.

7. References

1. Security in Clinical Information Systems, R.J. Anderson, published by the British Medical Association, January 1996.

2. An Update on the BMA Security Policy, R. Anderson, these Proceedings.

Privacy Oriented Clearing for the German Health-Care System

Gerrit Bleumer, Matthias Schunter
Universität Hildesheim, Institut für Informatik
Marienburger Platz 22, 31141 Hildesheim
{bleumer, schunter}@acm.org

Abstract. We present a clearing scheme for health-care in Germany that allows for the specific privacy interests of all participants, including the patient. Health insurance plays a key role in the German clearing system and it is their vital interest to reduce their overall cost as much as possible. Our scheme supports these interests while protecting the privacy of the insured persons and medical professionals.

1 Introduction

In most western democracies the increasing diversification of health-care providers and their ongoing competition enforce lean administration procedures including charging and accounting. However, simply simulating paper-based procedures by distributed computer systems will endanger the legitimate privacy interests of the participants. In this paper we show that charging, clearing and an effective control of the total remuneration of the health-care system are possible while privacy for all participants is provided.

Former and current paper-based procedures relied on much identifying patient data in order to ensure integrity. The applicable law on data protection limited the leakage of identifiable information only to the extent that getting hold of such data, transferring or storing it was relatively bothering. The inevitable consequence was that patients lacked privacy against all parties involved in their treatment but were slightly protected against outsiders since copying the paper documents is costly. This does not hold for digital documents. Therefore, the easier it is to acquire data illegitimately, the more need protection measures be integrated into the technical infrastructures themselves.

On the one hand, new technologies bear new potentials of surveillance and control (computer aided evaluation, medical data warehouses), on the other hand they also facilitate a new quality of security — including security of *all* participants — by avoiding the storage of large amounts of personal data in central places (chipcards, electronic wallets, and personal digital assistants with keyboard and display [21]). Health-care providers are about to invest millions into new communication and computing infrastructures. These investments will pay only if the technologies respect the actual legal regulations and if their implications are tolerated or at least accepted by all participants affected, e.g., patients, medical professionals, health insurances, etc. The G7 and some national initiatives [8] have stimulated such technologies, the topic has been suggested for further research to the Commission of the European Communities [2, 3] and, for example, specific solutions for the US market are under development [17, 18].

In order to derive an acceptable solution we state the (professional) duties and goals of each participant and then answer the key question:

Who needs which data in order to fulfil their duties and meet their goals?

Depending on the answer, we will select suitable technical and cryptographic measures to build our protocols. In comparison to existing solutions [23, 24], our protocols do not only provide integrity, but also full privacy to all participants.

2 Contractual Framework

We introduce the participants and business transactions of the German health-care system [1, 7, 16] with respect to charging and clearing of medical services. Afterwards we deduce the security interests of the participants involved.

The German health-care system[1] consists of five supply sectors [1, 9]. *Medical Outpatient Treatment* includes registered physicians (GPs) and specialists, e.g., dentists, who have their own independent practices. *Paramedical Outpatient Treatment* includes professionals allied to medicine like physio-therapists, speech therapists, etc. The *Inpatient Treatment* consists of all hospitals for acute cases and special hospitals. The *Public Health Services* are provided by state and local public health departments and by the departments of chemical examinations. The *Pharmaceutical Supply* is provided by pharmacists.

The health insurers are the clearing houses of the health-care system. In practice they delegate the clearing tasks to several client-specific organizations (*actual clearing houses*). There are compulsory and private health insurances. Roughly speaking, contributions to the former are income related, whereas those to the latter are risk-related. There is a level of income below which insurance is compulsory. The privacy interests of patients (and physicians) inherently conflict with the screening interests of private health insurers to such an extent that we suggest our solution for compulsory health insurers only. They pay about one half of the total cost in health-care.

Throughout this paper we distinguish three kinds of *health-care providers* (Fig. 1.) and draft their modes of charging.

1) Outpatient physicians registered by compulsory health insurers (*registered physicians*) may issue prescriptions for medical treatment and write letters of referral. They do not claim directly to the health insurers. Their actual clearing houses are the local associations of registered physicians: Kassenärztliche Vereinigungen (KV). Each KV gets a lump sum from the compulsory health insurers and reimburses the invoices of registered physicians. The registration is done by a joint registration committee of the health insurances and the KVs.
2) *Pharmacists* and *paramedical professionals* serve patients more or less according to what registered physicians have prescribed. Their actual clearing houses are the health insurers.
3) *Inpatient physicians*, analogously to outpatient physicians, do not claim directly to the health insurers. Their clearing houses are their respective hospitals which in turn are reimbursed by the health insurers.

3 Paper-based Charging and Clearing

We consider in more detail how expenses for medical treatment and medicaments are claimed in the German health-care system. Interactions between two participants consist

1) A German-English and English-German glossary about the German health-care system can be found in [1].

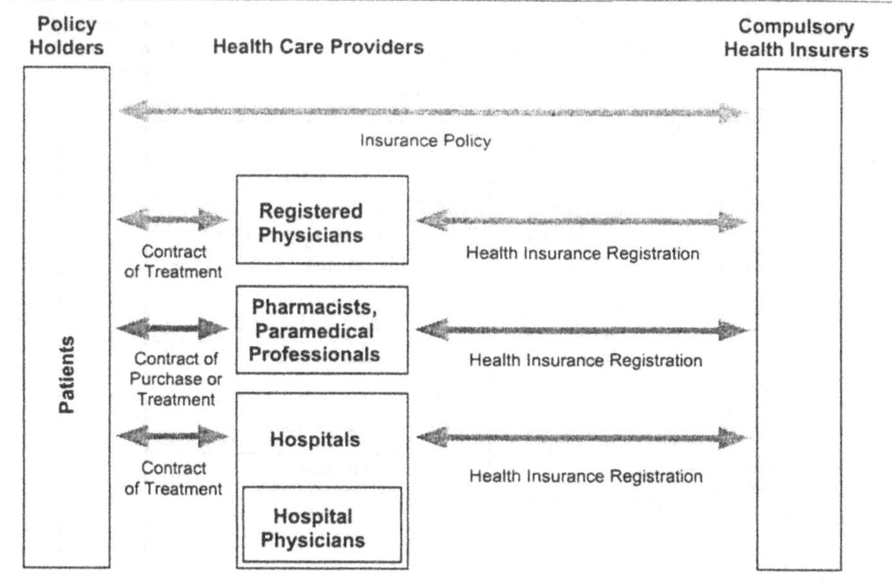

Fig. 1. Contractual Framework

of "real" actions and of "paper" actions. For example, a physician treats a patient, sends an invoice for the treatment and is finally refunded. We regard the first and last of these actions as "real" and the second as a paper action. Our focus is on electronic transactions substituting the paper actions, particularly those containing identifying patient data (Fig. 2.).

Consider a typical process of treatment: A patient requests treatment from his GP by handing over a signed health insurance record card (Krankenschein) and includes the data necessary for accounting. The GP may provide some treatment on his own and in addition:

1) prescribe some medicament, and
2) refer the patient to a specialist or hospital.

During the process of health-care, these steps can be iterated with various medical professionals taking responsibility for the patient and delegating it further. In each of the three cases, the GP produces a medical record that contains accounting data and possibly diagnostic, therapeutic or prognostic information about the patient. Usually, the patient passes a relevant excerpt of this record to the next health-care provider, who then continues the process of treatment. Each health-care provider copies the respective part of the patient's record and forwards it to the respective actual clearing house in order to legitimate his invoice.

3.1 Analysis

Since 1992 the compulsory health insurers have equipped their policy holders with personal health insurance cards ("Versichertenkarte"). These are memory chip cards containing the administrative data of a patient that had previously been communicated by a paper-based health insurance record card. If a patient requests a medical service from a health-

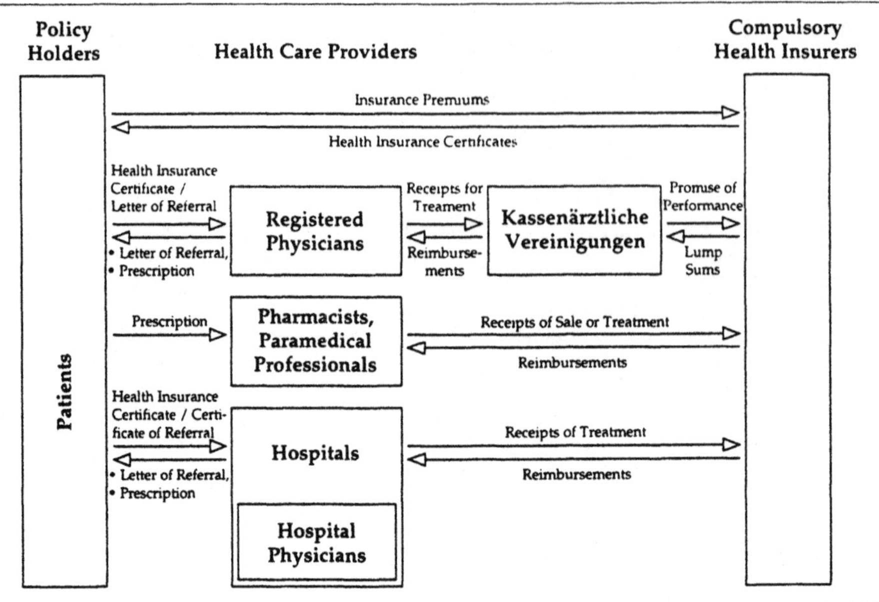

Fig. 2. Flow of Information Between the Participants of the German Health-care System

care provider, he has to identify himself by his health insurance card. Clearly, this is an almost perfect means to efficiently and reliably enforce the complete identification of patients — the primary requirement of health insurers. The privacy requirements of patients, however, have simply been ignored.

The paper-based refund system implements a kind of postpaid system. Forms for health insurance record cards can be regarded as special kinds of credit cards. Filling in such a form legitimates a patient to get, e.g., medical treatment. The health insurer of the patient acts as the clearing house. It pays lump sums to the actual clearing houses and these reimburse the expenses that are properly supported with receipts.

Alternatively, health-care providers could also claim directly to the patients, as most insurers do, e.g., private health or car insurances. In this case, policy holders get to know the detailed cost of their treatments and could act in a more cost-saving way. On the one hand, they could ask their health-care providers for less expensive services and could check all invoices. On the other hand, they could occasionally decide whether to use their health insurer or whether they like to pay by themselves.

Usually, receipts for everyday's commercial transactions do not contain much personal information about the payer; receipts in health-care are different. In paper-based systems the invoices of the health-care providers (and the receipts of the actual clearing houses) contain a tremendous amount of highly personal and sensitive information about patients and physicians. The mere existence of charging documents containing identifying information about patients tempts people to use this information for secondary purposes. Every participant involved gets to know the complete prescription for a patient and all documents referring to a patient are linked from the treating physician at the front end to the health insurer at the other end.

3.2 Participants and Their Specific Security Requirements

In order to motivate our alternative, we settle the question which participants really need to have which information in order to fulfil their tasks. We recall the services to be provided by each participant (Section 3.2.1) and consider additional constraints posed by the specific confidentiality and privacy needs of all participants (Section 3.2.2).

3.2.1 Availability and Integrity Requirements

Physician: Each patient shall receive exactly the treatment and medicament as is prescribed. In particular, each prescription shall be used at most once. In some cases an extended validity of prescriptions is required according to a therapy plan.

Policy holder: If he presents a valid health-insurance certificate, letter of referral, or prescription to a health-care provider of his choice, the provider shall indeed offer the requested service or perform the treatment prescribed.

Pharmacies and Paramedical professionals: Any of their expenses should be reimbursed by the health insurers if the health-care provider is registered and if the claims are properly supported by proofs of treatment.

Health insurers: Only registered physicians should be able issue prescriptions. Each policy holder should be able to use prescriptions at most once or according to a therapy plan, respectively. Each health insurer should reimburse expenses only once and only if they have been spent for its own policy holders. Health insurers should be able to limit the total reimbursement per year ("Deckelungsprinzip").

Clearly, the health-care providers usually need few administrative data of the patients they treat or sell medicine to. Even less administrative data about patients needs to be communicated between health-care providers. The patients need non-repudiable prescriptions of their physicians. The health service providers need to verify the prescriptions before giving any treatments or medicines. Afterwards, they need to obtain receipts for the services provided. In paper-based practice, the medical prescription serves for both purposes. What we learn from this summary is that the patients' real names need to be included only in their health insurance policies.

3.2.2 Confidentiality and Privacy Requirements

Physician and Patient: Medical treatment requires a relationship based on trust between patient and physician. Their relationship has to be protected comprehensively against third parties' interests; diagnoses and therapies should be strictly confidential. This specific rule should override, for example, a general obligation to escrow cryptographic keys. In general, health insurers do not need to know and thus should not know which physicians their policy holders visit.

Physician: At least by default, health insurers should not be able to monitor the physicians' habits to treat their patients and to prescribe medicaments. The interest and obligation of health insurers to save cost of health-care hardly justifies more control than spot-checking physicians.

Policy holder: The policy holder's right to ask a health-care provider of his choice for second opinions implies that different health-care providers should not monitor policy holders by exchanging their local views on them.

Obviously, the above requirements can be met by legal regulations, but technical means are more effective; even more so if they can be enforced by the policy holders themselves. Therefore, we introduce pseudonyms for policy holders as well as for physicians and we propose to employ them consistently in any charging interaction of physicians and policy holders [19, 20].

4 Digital Charging and Clearing Procedures

We now show how the whole process of treatment can be organized in a privacy-oriented way. The underlying idea is to use a modified prepay system rather than simulating the postpaid system of the paper world. Each health insurance maintains its own digital currency. The coins are labelled and represent Health Insurance certificates (***I*-certificates**), which legitimate for certain treatments (e.g., visiting a GP, dentist, etc.). Health-care providers maintain their own digital currency. These coins are also labelled and represent Medical certificates (***M*-certificates**) that we use as a generic term for prescriptions, letters of referral, etc. *M*-certificates can be issued such that they only reveal a group to which the actual issuer belongs — not the issuer himself. We assume that each policy holder is equipped with a personal user device [21] capable to manage his or her certificates and that each health-care provider offers appropriate stationary equipment to interact with personal devices. Note that this fulfilled by smartcards which will be introduced, except for a missing secure user interface.

4.1 Initialization

There are three initializing steps as illustrated in Fig. 3.. Since these steps are independent, they may be executed in any order.

<i> In order to facilitate their policy holders to receive treatment anonymously, each health insurer issues batches of *I*-certificates to its policy holders. *I*-certificates have the following properties:

a) From a given *I*-certificate one can determine the actual health insurer of a policy holder but learns nothing more about the holder's identity.

b) *I*-certificates can be used at most once. Using one twice in order to receive a service twice, reveals the policy holder's identity. Observe that copying an I-certificate is not prevented, but if the original owner would use it, too, the double-show detection mechanism will identify him.

<ii> Physicians can form groups that could be administered, e.g., by the respective KV or hospital. Members of a group can claim their expenses anonymously, i.e., relative to their group. Examples for such groups are the GPs of a geographical region, or the physicians of a hospital department. The size and structure of these groups is subject to balancing the monitoring interests of health insurers and the privacy interests of the physicians.

<iii> Each health-care provider has his specific signature key by which he signs his invoices later on. Health-care providers are registered by a committee of the health

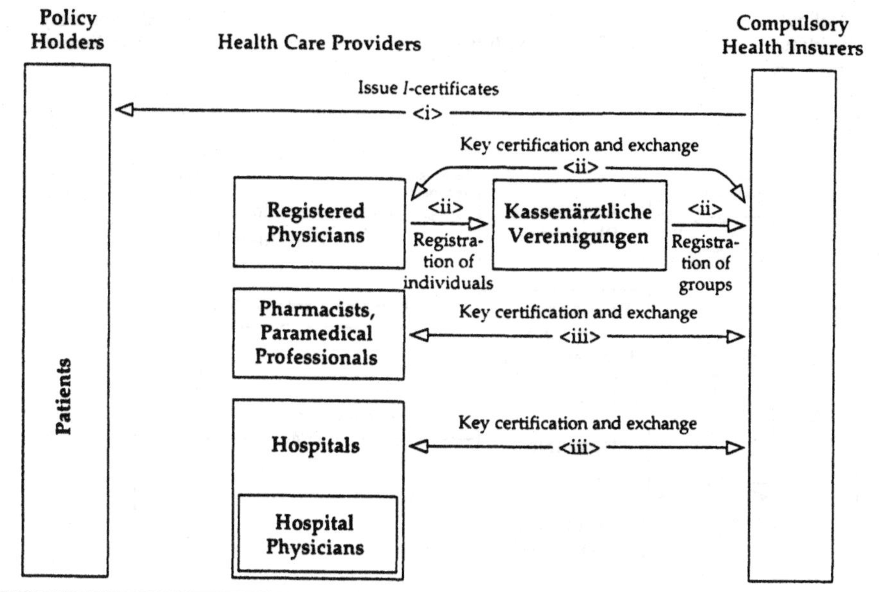

Fig. 3. Initialization

insurers by having their corresponding public keys registered. Alternatively, the committee may delegate this registration to the KV.

An overview over the stages of charging and clearing is shown in Fig. 4..

4.2 Issuing Prescriptions

<1> When a policy holder —now acting as a patient— is to receive a prescription, he pays a fresh *I*-certificate to his physician and gets a respective *M*-certificate in return. Physicians record all treatment and prescriptions they have provided to their patients.

4.3 Showing Prescriptions

<2> The patient shows a new *I*-certificate as a proof of being member of a health insurance together with the *M*-certificate received in order to show his prescription to an provider (e.g. a pharmacist). The provider checks both certificates and provides the prescribed treatment or medicament(s). In the next section we show how this can be implemented by means of one-show group credentials [4, 10].

4.4 Digital Clearing of Prescriptions

<3> The health-care provider sends the transcripts of the received certificates to the respective health insurer in order to prove his expenses. The health insurer checks the validity of the transcripts and checks for double showing. The health insurer also checks for the budgeting of the groups. If a group of health-care providers exceeds a certain budget, its group center can be asked to deanonymize some or all of the transcripts of a group to find out which provider(s) caused the trouble.

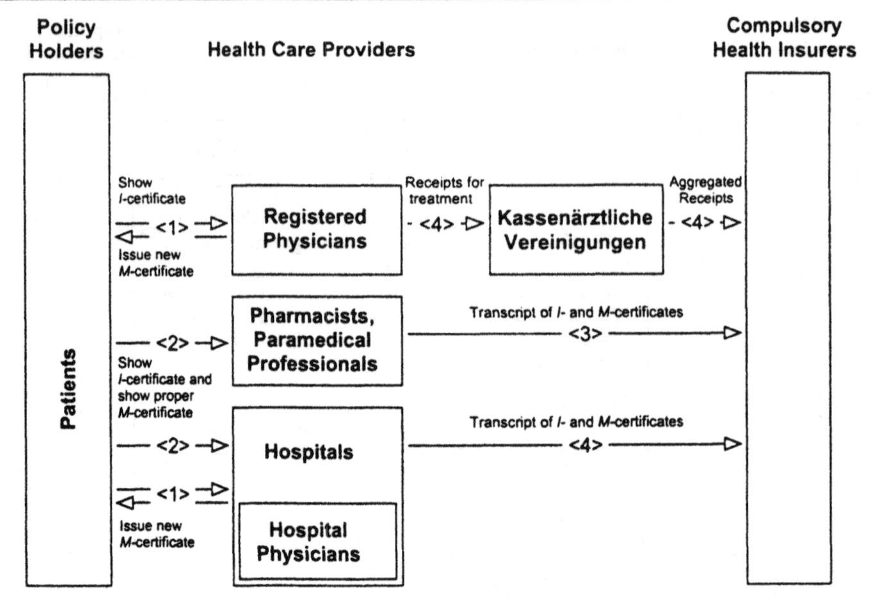

Fig. 4. Digital Charging of Medical Services.

The health-care providers need not trust the health insurers, because, if need be, the providers can prove all their claims to an arbiter or a court.

4.5 Digital Clearing of Medical Treatment

Different from pharmacists and paramedical professionals, physicians decide autonomously about therapies they perform or prescribe and thereby determine the amounts claimed. In the current paper-based system this autonomy is hardly controlled; even the compulsory insured patients cannot check if the expenses claimed correlate to the treatment they received. This can be implemented straightforwardly. Health insurers simply accept the transcripts of *M*-certificates containing the corresponding *I*-certificates as valid proof of treatment. If health insurers request more control, they could ask the physicians to have their invoices signed (anonymously) by their respective patients (see Section 3.1).

According to Section 3.2, we must consider the following requirements:

1) The trust relationship between physician and patient must be protected. Transcripts or combinations of transcripts resulting from this relationship (prescriptions, etc.) must not reveal the identity of physician or patient.
2) Exceptional rules must be supported because the physician in charge of a patient is ultimately responsible and liable for how the patient is treated and what he is told. For example, in case of an emergency, a physician's expenses must be reimbursed even if the patient is not able to confirm or consent to anything. Another case occurs when a physician decides not to tell the whole story to his patient.

A possible trade-off is the following:

<4> Patients confirm and sign the medical reports about their treatment. The physicians keep the signed reports with the patient's record. The physicians write anonymous invoices and claim to the respective KV or their employing hospital, e.g., every quarter of a year. After checking the budgets, all reimbursements are payed.

The physicians record the signed confirmations of their patients. If a health insurer detects that some budget is exceeded, it may ask for these confirmations. These confirmations may be signed anonymously (see Section 4.5) using a group signature scheme to protect the privacy of the patients even in the presence of extensive spot-checking. In addition, the KVs may spot-check physicians, i.e., ask for these confirmations of randomly selected patients, too.

4.6 Security

We explicate why the proposed solution meets the requirements described in Section 3.2:

4.6.1 Availability and Integrity Requirements

Physician: Each patient shall receive exactly the treatment and medicaments as is prescribed. In particular, each prescription shall be received once and only once. In some cases an extended validity of prescriptions is required according to a therapy plan.

Any modification of a M-certificate's label invalidates the certificate itself because it invalidates the digital signature involved in the cryptographic implementation of certificates. The one-time property of M-certificates ensures that each prescription can be used only once.

Policy holder: If he presents a valid health-insurance certificate, letter of referral, or prescription to a health-care provider of his choice, the provider shall indeed offer the requested service or perform the treatment prescribed.

The integrity requirement is met since the employed credential scheme is correct. The availability requirement cannot be enforced, it is "only" supported by the legal contract between health-care providers and health insurers: If a patient shows a valid prescription, the provider is obliged to provide the prescribed treatment.

Pharmacist and Paramedical professionals: Any of their expenses should be reimbursed by the health insurers if the health-care provider is registered and the expenses claimed are properly supported by proofs of treatment.

Providers use M-certificate transcripts as receipts to the health insurers. As M-certificates as well as their transcripts reveal a group of their issuer, health insurers can make sure to accept only M-certificates that have been issued by physicians.

Health insurers: Only registered physicians should be able issue prescriptions. Each policy holder should be able to use prescriptions at most once or according to a therapy plan, respectively. Each health insurer should reimburse expenses only once and only if they have been spent for its own policy holders. Health insurers should be able to limit the total reimbursement per year ("Deckelungsprinzip").

Registrations of physicians are checked in the same way as those of pharmacies and paramedical professionals. Showing prescriptions more than once will be recognized by the health insurers when performing a double show detection.

Reimbursement of expenses for own policy holders cannot be enforced strictly in the paper-based system. The same holds for our digital scheme: Two potential attackers need to be addressed, policy holders and non-policy holders, and collusions thereof. Non-policy holders could get hold of the personal user device of a policy holder and thus of his certificates. Potential damage of this attack could be limited by two measures: Each personal user device should identify its owner, e.g., by means of biometrics, and all critical operations should be protected by means of passwords, PINs, etc. More dangerously, policy holders could try to sell their certificates or their whole personal user devices together with passwords and PINs. This may be prevented by means of a printed photographs on the device. This kind of insurance fraud cannot be strictly prevented, but health insurers can limit the number of *I*-certificates issued just like banks do with usual checks.

The total reimbursement per year can be controlled by monitoring and budgeting the groups of physicians.

4.6.2 Privacy Requirements

Physician and Patient: Medical treatment requires a relationship based on trust between patient and physician. This relationship should be protected comprehensively against third parties' interests; diagnoses, therapies and prognoses should be strictly private. This specific rule should override, for example, a general obligation to escrow cryptographic keys. In general, health insurers do not need to know and thus should not know which physicians their policy holders visit.

Physicians achieve their privacy by charging and prescribing anonymously relative to one of their groups, and patients enforce their privacy by using a fresh certificate for every transaction. This combination guarantees that no participant other than the patient and the physician can link any two of their visits.

Physician: At least by default, health insurers should not be able to monitor the physicians' habits to treat their patients or to prescribe medicaments. The interest and obligation of health insurers to save cost of health-care hardly justifies more control than spot checking physicians.

In our proposal, the health insurers can profile only groups of physicians, not individual physicians.

Policy holder: The policy holder's right to ask a health-care provider of his choice for second opinions implies that different health-care providers should not monitor policy holders by exchanging their local views on them.

Since the patient uses a fresh pseudonym for each transaction, no two of his transactions can be linked (from the data he provides himself). This feature is supported by the personal user devices being indistinguishable on the network, e.g., no machine readable serial numbers must be present.

5 Implementing the Clearing Process

We show how to implement the clearing process described in Section 4 by four primitive schemes. The primitive schemes are introduced in Section 5.1, an implementation of the clearing process is sketched in Section 5.2 and the means to control cost are revisited in Section 5.2.9.

5.1 Primitive Schemes

We employ four primitive schemes: *ordinary digital signatures* (Section 5.1.1), *one-show credentials* (also called digital cash, Section 5.1.2). *group signatures* (Section 5.1.3) and *one-show group credentials* (Section 5.1.4). Each of these schemes has its own set of operations and security features. In order to indicate how the operations are going to be applied, we introduce them by referring to the now familiar participants: Health insurer (*H*), physician (*D*), pharmacist or paramedical professional (*E*) and policy holder (*P*). Some operations are to be implemented by two party protocols. In this case the last parameter of the formal parameter list of the operation is an address of the peer party.

5.1.1 Ordinary Digital Signatures

An ordinary digital signature under a message achieves non-repudiation of origin for the recipient of the message [15, 22]. An ordinary digital signature can be checked by anybody and, thus, can provide legal evidence for authorship of a message. The primitive offers three operations:

Generating Keys

Everyone who has a need to sign can generate a *private key* (*rk*) and a corresponding public key (*pk*). The private key is used to sign digital messages. The public key needs to be distributed in an authentic way, for example, by means of trust centers, and enables to test ordinary digital signatures. Everyone holding a signed message and the public key of the claimed signer can test whether the signature is valid or not.

$$(rk, pk) = \text{genKey}(\bullet)$$ [2]

Signing

Someone who has generated a private key can later sign a message m and obtain a signature σ.

$$\sigma = \text{sign}(rk, m)$$

Testing

Everyone can test the signature σ on message m by looking up the public key pk of the claimed signer.

$$ok = \text{test}(pk, \sigma, m)$$

5.1.2 One-Show Credentials

A one-show credential scheme (also called digital cash scheme) provides the digital analogue of coins of some currency [5, 6, 11]. Credentials reveal the identity of their issuer, e.g., a health insurer, but keep the holder anonymous against both the issuer and the recipient to whom the credential is shown. A credential can be checked by anybody and, thus, can provide legal evidence for an authorization of the holder. The primitive offers five operations:

---

2) All key generating operations are probabilistic algorithms, so that their outcome cannot be predicted. The bullet in the parameter list is a place holder for one or more security parameters, which are not important in this context.

Generating Keys

The health insurer H, which has to issue some kind of currency, can generate a *private key* (rk) and a corresponding public key (pk). The private key is used to create and issue credentials. The public key needs to be distributed just as for ordinary digital signatures, and enables to check credentials.

$$(rk, pk) = \text{genKeyCred}(\bullet)$$

Issuing Credentials

A health insurer H with private key rk_H issues a credential labelled with a type identifier l to a policy holder P. The result is a one-show credential I, which later represents an I-certificate:

$$I = \text{issue}(rk_H, l, P)$$

Showing Credentials

Having received a credential I, a policy holder P can show it to some physician D. D checks the credential by using the public key pk of the claimed issuer I. If physician D accepts the credential, he ends up with a transcript t_I that he uses later to deposit the received credential.

$$t_I = \text{show}(pk_H, I, D)$$

Depositing Credentials

A physician D who has received a credential I proves this fact to an insurer H by providing a transcript t_I. The insurer checks the validity of t_I by using the insurer's public key pk_H.

$$ok = \text{deposit}(pk_H, t_I, H)$$

Double Showing Detection

As an integral part of checking the validity of a transcript, the health insurer checks if the credential has been spent and claimed previously. If so, the insurer can determine the identity of the policy holder who once received that credential. This requires only the two different transcripts t_I, t_I' that resulted from showing the credential twice. The parameter list contains the actual transcript t_I and the history of all transcripts deposited before (indicated by •)

$$id = \text{identifyShower}(t_I, \bullet)$$

Instead of detecting double-showers after the fact, such fraud can also be prevented by using wallets with observer for the user devices [12]. Double deposits of an identical transcript are usually prevented by randomizing the signatures and rejecting the second deposit after showing the first signature.

5.1.3 Group Signatures

Group Signatures [12, 14] can be regarded as anonymous ordinary digital signatures. Signers can dynamically form groups and sign in behalf of their group(s). Each group publishes a public group key by which outsiders can test whether a signature originates from a member of that group, but not from whom. However, a group signature contains enough information to identify the actual signer if a dispute arises later on. A dedicated center in each group could manage registration and suspension of members as well as re-identifications. The primitive offers five operations:

Generating Keys and Managing Groups

Every physician D who has a need to sign anonymously can generate a private individual key (ri_D) and corresponding public individual key pi_D:

$$(ri_D, pi_D) = \text{genIKey}(\bullet)$$

Registration as a member of a group G is done by handing over one's public individual key and receiving the public group key pk_G in return. (The public individual keys are known by the respective group center(s) only, not by the general public.) In addition, the group center maintains a private group key rk_G that is used for identification of group members only (The public individual keys of all group members are one input to this procedure.):

$$(rk_G, pk_G) = \text{genGKey}(\bullet)$$

Signing

A member D of group G can sign a message m anonymously on input her or his private and public individual keys and the group's public key. The following group signature is obtained:

$$\sigma = \text{gSign}(ri_D, pi_D, pk_G, m)$$

Testing

Everyone can test a signature σ on message m by looking up the public key pk_G of the group G by what the message is claimed to be signed. A positive result assures the verifier that the signer is a member of group G, but gives no further indication who the signer is.

$$ok = \text{gTest}(pk_G, \sigma, m)$$

Identifying

Given a message m signed by a member D of group G, the center of G can identify the signer by determining his public individual key:

$$pi = \text{identifySigner}(rk_G, pk_G, \sigma, m)$$

5.1.4 One-Show Group Credentials

This primitive extends one-show credentials in much the same way as group signature schemes extend ordinary digital signature schemes. Group credentials do not reveal their actual issuer, but only a group to which the issuer is registered. In case of a dispute, the actual issuer can later be identified by the center of the respective group. Group credentials offer seven operations:

Generating Keys and Managing Groups

Every physician D who has a need to issue group credentials can generate a pair of individual keys, a private (ri_{pD}) and corresponding public one pi_D:

$$(ri_D, pi_D) = \text{genIKeyCred}(\bullet)$$

Registration as a member of a group G is done by handing over one's public individual key and receiving for it the public group key pk_G in return. In addition, the group center maintains a private group key rk_G that is used for identification of group members only:

$$(rk_G, pk_G) = \text{genGKeyCred}(\bullet)$$

Issuing Group Credentials

A physician D registered as a member of group G issues a credential labelled l to a policy holder P. The result is a one-show group credential M, later representing an M-certificate:

$$M = \text{gIssue}(ri_D, pi_D, pk_G, l, P)$$

Showing Group Credentials

Having received a group credential M, a policy holder P can show it to some physician D. D checks the credential by using the public key pk_G of the claimed issuer group. If physician D accepts the credential, he ends up with a transcript t_M that he uses later to deposit the received credential and get reimbursed.

$$t_M = \text{gShow}(pk_G, M, D)$$

Depositing Group Credentials

A physician D who has received a group credential M proves this fact to an insurer H by providing a transcript t_M. The insurer H checks the validity of t_M by using the public key pk_G of the group G of the issuer.

$$ok = \text{gDeposit}(pk_G, t_M, H)$$

Identifying Issuers

Given a group credential M issued by any of the members of group G, the center of G can identify the issuer D by determining his public individual key:

$$pi_D = \text{identifyIssuer}(rk_G, pk_G, M)$$

Double Showing Detection

As an integral part of checking the validity of a transcript, the health insurer checks if the credential has been shown or deposited before. If so, the insurer can determine the identity of the policy holder who once received that credential. This requires only the two different transcripts t_M, t_M' that resulted from showing the credential twice. The parameter list contains the actual transcript t_M, and the history of all transcripts deposited before (indicated by •):

$$id = \text{gIdentifyShower}(t_M, \bullet)$$

5.2 Draft Protocols

The idea underlying our proposal is to implement I-certificates by one-show credentials (depicted as white coins in the following figures) and M-certificates by one-show group credentials (depicted as shaded coins). In order to sign their invoices, physicians use group signatures and all other health-care providers use ordinary digital signatures.

We are going to walk through a complete charging and clearing example including one health insurer H, one of its policy holders P, a physician D and a pharmacist or paramedical professional E. Each step is implemented by means of the primitives of Section 5.1. The initialization phase is depicted in Fig. 5. (Section 5.2.1 through 5.2.4). The subsequent actions for charging and clearing of medical treatment and accounting are depicted in Fig. 6. (Section 5.2.5 through 5.2.8).

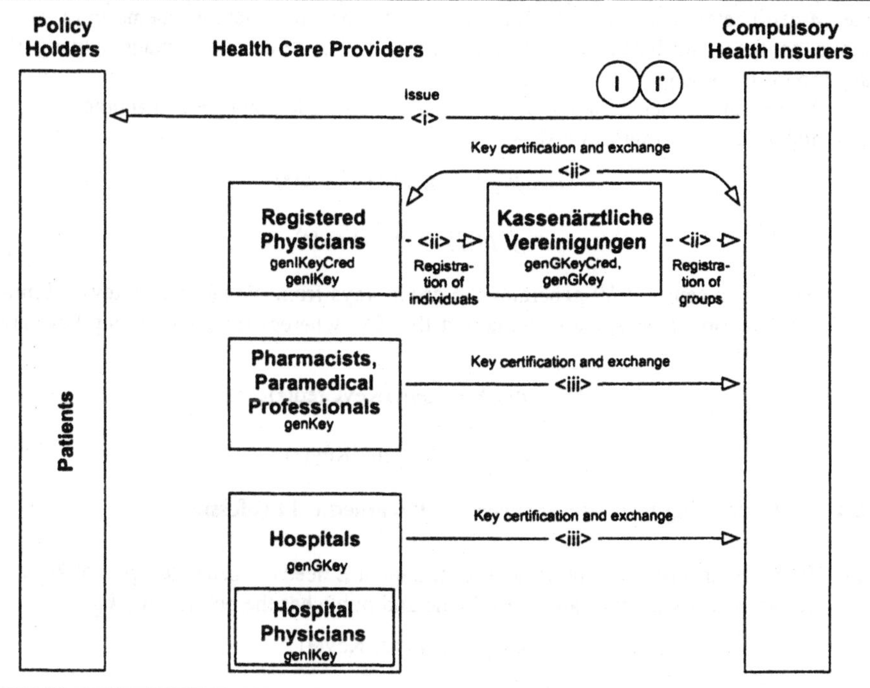

Fig. 5. Initialization Phase

5.2.1 Initialization

Physicians have to generate a pair of individual keys for a group signature scheme and one for a group credential scheme. The former is to claim the expenses for their medical treatment, the latter is to issue prescriptions to their patients. Pharmacies and paramedical professionals have to generate an individual pair of keys for an ordinary digital signature scheme.

5.2.2 Generating Health Insurance Record Cards

Health insurers issue batches of one-time credentials to their policy holders. For every health insurance record card a policy holder needs, he uses a fresh credential later on (Section 5.1.4).

<i> A health insurer using private key rk_H issues to its policy holder P a batch of credentials that facilitate to visit a GP:

$$(I, I', \ldots) = \text{issue}(rk_H, \text{'GP'}, P)$$

5.2.3 Generating Provider Licenses for Medical Professions

Before physicians can issue prescription or claim expenses for medical treatment, they have to be registered to respective groups of physicians. These groups could be managed, e.g., by the KVs. Registration to a physicians' group serves as a legitimation to claim expenses for medical treatment to a health insurer and, thus, is an analogue to provider licenses of physicians. Registration is by generating two individual keys and having their public parts registered by the group center. One is of a group credential scheme in order to issue M-certificates (Section 5.1.4), the other is of a group signature scheme in order to claim expenses for medical treatment (Section 5.1.3). We see no disadvantage in using the same groups for both purposes:

<ii> Physician D generates a pair of individual group credential keys and another pair of individual group signature keys:

$$(ri_D, pi_D) = \text{genIKeyCred}(\bullet)$$

$$(ri_D', pi_D') = \text{genIKey}(\bullet)$$

The group center (KV) generates the group keys from the individual keys submitted. The private group keys remain at the KV, whereas the public group keys are published:

$$(rk_G, pk_G) = \text{genGKeyCred}(\bullet).$$

$$(rk_G', pk_G') = \text{genGKey}(\bullet)$$

5.2.4 Generating Provider Licenses for Paramedical Professionals

<ii> Each pharmacist and paramedical professional E needs to generate a pair of keys for an ordinary digital signature scheme and publishes the public key pk_E:

$$(rk_E, pk_E) = \text{genKey}(\bullet)$$

Fig. 6. illustrates the processes of issuing prescriptions, charging medicaments and medical treatment.

5.2.5 Issuing a Prescription

<1> After examining his patient P, physician D can issue a prescription m to P by means of a one-show group credential M:

$$M = \text{gIssue}(ri_D, pi_D, pk_G, m, P),$$

5.2.6 Showing a Prescription

<2> Patient P who has received a group credential M can show it to a pharmacist or paramedical professional E. In addition, he shows a fresh credential Γ in order to prove his membership in a health insurance. If E accepts, he is left with two transcripts t_Γ and t_M.

$$t_\Gamma = \text{show}(pk_H, \Gamma, E), \quad t_M = \text{gShow}(pk_G, M, E)$$

If a patient shows the same (group) credential twice, the fraud will be detected at clearing time. If, for example, duplicate delivery of drugs is to be prevented, the pharmacy needs to check on-line whether the M-certificate has been shown before.

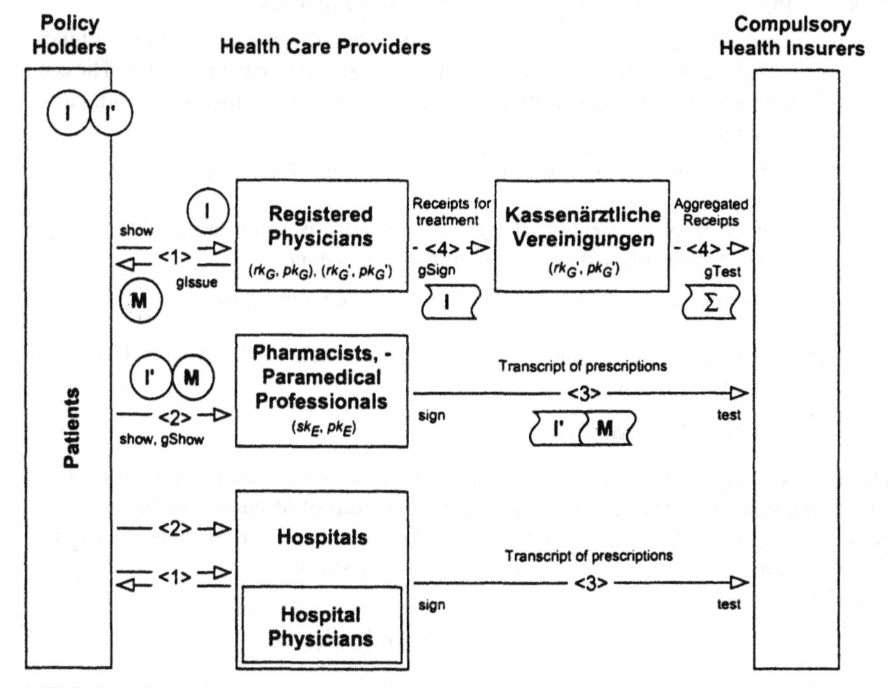

Fig. 6. Charging Medical Treatment and Prescriptions and Clearing

5.2.7 Depositing Prescriptions on Health Insurers' Accounts

<3> A pharmacist or paramedical professional E claims his expenses for a prescribed service m to the respective health insurer H by forwarding his signed invoice including both the credential transcript (I-certificate) and the group credential transcript (M-certificate):

$$\sigma = \text{sign}(rk_E, (\text{invoice}, t_{I'}, t_M)),$$

$$ok = \text{deposit}(pk_H, t_{I'}, H)$$

$$ok = \text{gDeposit}(pk_G, t_M, H)$$

The health insurer accepts if the signature is valid and the double show detection fails for both transcripts:

$$ok = \text{test}(pk_E, \sigma, (\text{invoice}, t_{I'}, t_M)),$$

$$\text{identifyShower}(t_{I'}, \bullet),$$

$$\text{gIdentifyShower}(t_M, \bullet)$$

Recall that prescriptions of risky or expensive medicaments like drugs that should not be delivered twice for one prescription require double show prevention after step <2> already.

5.2.8 Placing Medical Treatment on the Account of a KV

<4> A physician D claims his expenses for medical treatment m to a KV in a similar way as pharmacists and paramedical professionals do to health insurers. The only difference is that physicians confirm their treatments anonymously by using a group signature:

$$\sigma = \mathrm{gSign}(ri_D, pi_D, pk_G, (\mathrm{invoice}, t_\Gamma)), \quad ok = \mathrm{deposit}(pk_G, t_\Gamma, H)$$

The health insurer accepts if the group signature is valid and no double-deposit occurred. Afterwards, a double-spending check is done:

$$ok = \mathrm{gTest}(pk_G, \sigma, (\mathrm{invoice}, t_\Gamma)), \quad \mathrm{identifyShower}(t_\Gamma, \bullet)$$

If the health insurer is not willing to bear the risk of double-spending, on-line checks must be mandatory.

5.2.9 Limiting the Total Cost

The above concept of charging and clearing enables the health insurers to limit the overall cost of the system. Health insurers can monitor the sum of M-certificates issued by each group of physicians. If certain groups exceed their budget, the KVs or hospitals can be asked to identify those physicians issuing significantly above average:
<3> KVs:

$$D = \mathrm{identifyIssuer}(rk_G, pk_G, M)$$

Furthermore, the KVs could recommend practices for subsequent spot-checking.

The health insurers can also limit the cost of medical services. The expenses claimed by pharmacies and paramedical professionals can be monitored individually. Those of physicians can be monitored with respect to the groups maintained. Health-care providers who have over-claimed can be identified similar as above.
<3> KVs:

$$D = \mathrm{identifySigner}(rk_G, pk_G, \sigma, m)$$

The health insurers can coarsely limit the overall cost by limiting the amount of I-certificates they issue. If a certain overall limit L per year must not be exceeded at all, any cost could be claimed in a virtual currency. At the end of a year the value of a unit of this virtual currency is calculated and all health-care providers are reimbursed according to this actual exchange rate. In addition, a small percentage of policy holders might be asked to participate in cross-section studies, etc.

6 Conclusions

We have shown that charging and clearing in the German health-care system can be done while the security and privacy interests of all participants and, particularly, of the patient-physician relation are respected. The proposal should be transferable to clearing systems of other solidarity-based reimbursement systems.

7 Acknowledgments

This work has been supported by many parties. We would like to thank the working group on security in hospital information systems of the German GMDS and in particular Bernd

Blobel and Klaus Pommerening for their motivation and support of this work. We have further appreciated the constructive criticism of Birgit Pfitzmann, Joachim Biskup and Simon Jenkins. This work has partially been supported by the German Research Foundation (DFG) and by the Commission of the European Union through their project SEMPER (Secure Electronic MarketPlace for EuRope).

8 References

[1] Arnold M, Brauer HP, Deneke V, Fiedler E: The Medical Profession in the Federal Republic of Germany; Deutscher Ärzte-Verlag, Köln-Lövenich 1982.

[2] Biskup J: Medical Database Security; Data Protection and Confidentiality in Health Informatics – Handling Health Data in Europe in the Future, Edited by the Commission of the European Communities DG XIII/F AIM, Proc. of the AIM Working Conference, Brussels, 19-21 March 1990, IOS Press, Amsterdam 1991, 214-230.

[3] Biskup J: Protection of privacy and confidentiality in medical information systems; Database Security, III: Status and Prospects (eds.: Spooner DL, Landwehr CE), North-Holland, 1990, 13 - 23.

[4] Bleumer G: Group Credentials; Hildesheimer Informatik Bericht (to appear in July 1996).

[5] Brands S: An Efficient Off-line Electronic Cash System Based On The Representation Problem; Centrum voor Wiskunde en Informatica, Computer Science/Departement of Algorithmics and Architecture, Report CS-R9323, March 1993.

[6] Brands S: Untraceable Off-line Cash in Wallet with Observers; Crypto '93, LNCS 773, Springer-Verlag, Berlin 1994 302-318.

[7] Buchholz EH: Unser Gesundheitswesen: Ein einführender Überblick zum Gesundheitswesen der Bundesrepublik Deutschland, Springer-Verlag, Berlin, 1988.

[8] Bundesministerium für Bildung, Wissenschaft, Forschung und Technologie: INFORMATIONSGESELLSCHAFT: Chancen, Innovationen und Herausforderungen; Rat für Forschung, Technologie und Innovation, Bundesministerium für Bildung, Wissenschaft, Forschung und Technologie, 1995.

[9] Bundesamt für Sicherheit in der Informationstechnik: Chipkarten im Gesundheitswesen; Schriftenreihe zur IT-Sicherheit Band 5, Bundesanzeiger Verlag, Köln 1995.

[10] Chaum D: Showing credentials without identification: Transferring signatures between unconditionally unlinkable pseudonyms; AUSCRYPT'90, Sydney, Australia, January 1990, LNCS 453, Springer-Verlag, Berlin 1990, 246-264.

[11] Chaum D, Fiat A, Naor M: Untraceable Electronic Cash, Crypto '88, LNCS 403, Springer-Verlag, Berlin 1990, 319-327.

[12] Chaum D, van Heijst E: Group Signatures; Eurocrypt '91, LNCS 547, Springer-Verlag, Berlin 1991, 257-265.

[13] Chaum D, Pedersen TP: Wallet Databases with Observers; Crypto '92, LNCS 740, Springer Verlag, Berlin 1993, 89-105.

[14] Chen L, Pedersen TP: New Group Signature Schemes; EUROCRYPT '94, Proceedings, LNCS 950, Springer-Verlag, Berlin 1995, 171-181.

[15] Diffie W, Hellman ME: New Directions in Cryptography; IEEE Transactions on Information Theory 22/6 (1976) 644-654.

[16] Häußler S, Liebold R, Narr H: Die Kassenärztliche Tätigkeit; Springer-Verlag, Berlin, 1984.

[17] Low SH, Maxemchuk NF: Anonymous Credit Cards; 2nd ACM Conference on Computer and Communications Security, Fairfax, November 1994, ACM Press, New York 1994, 108-117.

[18] Maxemchuk NF, Low SH: The Use of Communication Networks to Increase Personel Privacy in a Health Insurance Architecture; Manuscript, 1995

[19] Pommerening K, Pseudonyme - ein Kompromiß zwischen Anonymisierung und Personenbezug; in: Trampisch HJ, Lange S (Hrsg.): Medizinische Forschung — Ärztliches Handeln; 40. Jahrestagung der GMDS, Bochum, September 1995, MMV Medizin Verlag, München 1995, 329-333.

[20] Pommerening K: Chipkarten und Pseudonyme; F!FF Kommunikation 1/96, 9-12.

[21] Pfitzmann A, Pfitzmann B, Schunter M, Waidner M: Vertrauenswürdiger Entwurf portabler Benutzerendgeräte und Sicherheitsmodule; Brüggemann HH, Gerhardt-Häckl W (ed.): Verläßliche IT-Systeme, Proceedings der GI-Fachtagung VIS'95; DuD Fachbeiträge, Vieweg, Wiesbaden 1995, 329-350.

[22] Rivest RL, Shamir A, Adleman L: A Method for Obtaining Digital Signatures and Public-Key Cryptosystems; Communications of the ACM 21/2 (1978) 120-126, reprinted: 26/1 (1983) 96-99.

[23] Struif B: Das elektronische Rezept mit digitaler Unterschrift; Reimer H, Struif B (eds.): Kommunikation & Sicherheit, TeleTrust Deutschland e.V., Darmstadt 1992, 71-75.

[24] Struif B: Sicherheit und Datenschutz bei elektronischen Rezepten; Multicard'94, Elektronische Kartensysteme - Anspruch und Wirklichkeit, Kongreßdokument I, 23.-25. Februar 1994, Berlin, 71-80.

Personal Health Data on Optical Memory Cards in Isehara City

Yoshikazu OKADA, Yasuo HARUKI, Youich OGUSHI, Masanobu HORIE

School of Medicine, University of Tokai
Isehara, Kanagawa, JAPAN 259-11

1 Introduction

About 2,800 optical memory cards with personal health and welfare data have been at work in Isehara city (pop. 98,119 (1995)) since 1992. The card contains mainly the patient's basic personal health data including records of consultations for up to five years, the period stipulated in Japanese law. In some cases, the card may contain more data: examples include welfare data and medical images.

Even though the system has a software security mechanism, we think it important that holders can look at and maintain their data on their cards.

2 Short history of optical memory cards in Isehara city

The optical memory card system with health and welfare data was begun since 1992 with the cooperation of Isehara local government, Isehara medical association and Tokai university school of medicine, supported by the national government of Japan.

Now the system has 2,775 card holders and 24 terminals. The holders are mainly people over 65 years, because the system is based on the Japanese social health provision for older people. The potential number of users is about 9,000.

The terminals are situated in hospitals, clinics, a pharmacy, welfare centers and the city office. These terminals cover almost all the health and welfare facilities in Isehara city that older people habitually use. Although each card contains five years' consultation records and some contain welfare data and medical images, we estimate the optical card's capacity can also contain the important life-long record of the patient's health and welfare.

3 Data on the optical card

There are five groups of data on the card.

1. Basic information of the holder

2. Emergency data (blood type, allergic substances, etc.)
3. Results of physical examinations
4. History of welfare services
5. Medical records including medical images

All of these records are backed up in the appropriate institutions. For example, the records of consultations are stored in a database at the city office. The structure and function of each record is explained to the card owners by the providers, and they have full access to their records.

4 Security mechanism of the system

Each optical card is kept by its owner, who can control when and where to use it. The system also has three kinds of technical security mechanism.

4.1 Password

Each optical card has a four digit password, which is required to access the data on it.

4.2 Access card

Each health or welfare provider has another optical card that contains four digit passwords to access data on the customer's card. The system has 22 categories of provider (card owner, physician, public nurse, etc.), 352 categories of data, and three kinds of access method (read/write, read, none).

The data access granted to providers are restricted by their professions.

4.3 Owner's photograph

Each optical card stores the owner's portrait, which is displayed first when accessing the data on the card. This the provider can check that the holder has presented the right card.

4.4 Other features related to security

There are two optional security features:

1. Internal password — the user can define a password of up to 32 digits for every section of data on the card when the section is initialised. The password cannot be changed later.
2. Encryption — the optical card system can have encrypted data on it.

5 Automatic measurement and recording of blood pressure

We have implemented an automatic system for measuring and recording blood pressure since April 1996, in the Isehara city office. The system contains a PC, an optical card reader/writer and an automatic blood pressure meter.

5.1 Features

The card holders can insert their card in the card reader and can display a history of their blood pressure. Then they can press a button on the PC, whereupon the blood pressure meter begins a measurement and sends the result to the PC. The PC can display the new data and write them on to the card.

5.2 Data files

The system displays blood pressure data from health centers and from automatic blood pressure meters, and can write data only in a new section of the card. It can also maintain consistency of healthcare provider data and data collected by the card holder.

6 Discussion and Future plan

6.1 Features not in use

The optional passwords and data encryption are not used at present, because the system has only 24 terminals and we can control all the providers who use it. Our trial has shown that the system achieves an acceptable level of privacy.

6.2 Planned expansion

We now plan to expand the system to cope with more owners and more information on the card. Uses will include not just senior citizens but also ante- and post-natal clinics, student health, and the health of workers. The terminals will spread to a number of Japanese cities.

We plan to change the card data from fixed format to SGML (Standard General Markup Language). We may also use encryption technology for the new system.

6.3 Effects of patients writing data on the card

We plan to expand the range of health measurements that card holders can record on their cards by themselves. We feel that this will motivate the holders to be conscious of their health status. They should also notice the security system and derive confidence from it.

We think it is important to maintain privacy, and to make both card holders and health care providers conscious of it.

The Perspective of Medical Ethics

Dr. Fleur Fisher

Head of Ethics, Science and Information Division
British Medical Association

The concept of the confidentiality of the medical consultation has until very recently been believed to have the inviolability of the confessional. That the development of information technology, team working, and the financial contract between purchaser and provider organisations now threaten to destroy this confidentiality in the UK is the emotional equivalent of recognising that the confessional box is bugged.

The Western medical ethic, developed from the Greek tradition, has been built on the philosophy of the Hippocratic school.

> Into whatever houses I enter, I will go into them for the benefit of the sick, and will abstain from every voluntary act of mischief and corruption; and, further, from the seduction of females, or males, of freemen or slaves. Whatever, in connection with my professional practice, not in connection with it, I see or hear, in the life of men, which ought not to be spoken of abroad, I will not divulge, as reckoning that all such should be kept secret.

His concern for ethical behaviour was allied with a concern for the careful observation and scientific study of the disease. Later the Judeo-Christian influence on medical ethics derived from Jewish law administered by priests. As a nation fighting for survival, it was accepted that individual rights could be sacrificed for the community good — much of this was attention to effective public health measures. As Mason & McCall Smith point out in their standard UK text *Law and Medical Ethics*, this same group lifestyle with concepts of equality, charity and devotion to the less fortunate was a feature of the early Christian community and was kept alive through the Dark Ages through the infirmaries of the monasteries, the forerunners of hospitals.

The explosion of scientific thought and discovery in the 18th century threw up a galaxy of medical men and philosophers who accorded serious considerations to the essentials of the patient-physician contract, seized by the state of medical ethics (which had virtually degenerated to expression of medical etiquette and socially acceptable behaviour for doctors).

As Horner remarks in his thesis *Medical Ethics and Medical Practice*, similarities with the worldwide ethical dilemmas for doctors in our own time are striking.

Thomas Beddoes (1760–1808) was distressed by the profiteering from a gullible public by the rogues gallery of quacks peddling unproven cures. However, he found the profession little better than the quacks, and wrote that

> "medicine could be moved by money or it could be animated and organised by science, by the imperative search for truth"

He also opined that "informed choice is a myth".

Amongst these influential thinkers, John Gregory (1724-1773), often termed the first modern figure in Anglo American medical ethics was influenced by both David Hume and Adam Smith, whom he knew. He described medicine as "the art of preserving health, of prolonging life, of curing diseases" and wrote about the confidentiality of the consultation as well as listening to the patient, truthfulness in the face of uncertainty, and he believed that the physician should never abandon hopeless cases. Sympathy with the patient, humanity, gentleness of manners and a compassionate heart he deemed essential for a doctor.

The Utilitarian philosophies of Jeremy Bentham and John Stuart Mill were energetically opposed by a leading Anglican, Thomas Gisborne, who in 1794 produced a best-seller *An Enquiry into the Duties of Men in the Higher and Middle Classes of Society in Great Britain, Resulting from their Respective Stations, Professions and Employments*, which ran to six editions in seventeen years, becoming the popular text guiding ethical professional behaviour. He paid particular attention to unethical aspects of the practice of medicine, criticising the "sick trade".

Thomas Percival (1740-1804) often characterised as the father of modern medical ethics was the intellectual child of the political and social tumult of his times. Percival is in the tradition of "virtue ethics", drawing on Gisborne's concept of a social contract, i.e. he believed that groups or individuals given privileges by society must accept equivalent duties and responsibilities. He saw the physician as a quasi public servant. He considered that doctors *must* make ethical judgements, and contributed to the idea of the collective norm of behaviour and competence of the profession. He first proposed that patients with grievances be referred to present them to the faculty for resolution — the profession thus being seen to have a collective responsibility for its members. In 1847 the American Medical Association adopted a code of ethics based on Percival's work, with confidentiality and respect for the patient being among its fundamental principles.

Thus the unique relationship has historically been built on a foundation of trust. It is a one to one relationship. The doctors' overriding responsibility is to their patient, and as a professional the doctor strives at all times to protect that relationship — even at personal cost. Though political systems change this principle is the continuing thread that binds doctors together both down the centuries and across cultures.

The responsibility of the profession for its contact with society — a duty to ensure competence and adherence to the historical ethic of the doctor patient relationship — were important elements in the early years of what later became the British Medical Association (some of this has been categorised as protecting not only the honour but the income of the profession)!

In 1832 the Provincial Medical & Surgical Association (later the BMA) held its inaugural meeting Worcester when its founder, Charles Hastings, first referred to "the medical profession". By 1838 the Association produced a report for Council on the "evils of quackery" in which the need for registration and statutory regulation was recognised. At that time there were 21 ways in which one could be authorised to practice medicine, including recommendation by the Archbishop of Canterbury. The 1841 census records 33,339 people practising medicine, about 3 times the number of qualified practitioners recorded a decade later. By 1858 a Medical Act was passed. It was 1880 before an effective body for regulation was in place, however. The main objectives of reform were:

1. legal definition of qualified medical practitioners;
2. annually published register of all legally qualified medical practitioners;
3. for it to be a legal offence to describe oneself as a medical practitioner unless on the register;
4. to erase practitioners "guilty of certain disgraceful offences" from the register;
5. that doctors could practice anywhere in the UK.

There have been further medical acts. In 1978 the BMA's Central Ethical Committee voted that the General Medical Council give guidance for members of the medical profession on standards of professional conduct or on medical ethics. The Medical Act 1978 (in force from August 1980) confirmed this.

And in 1983 the General Medical Council brought out its book, first of a series *Professional Conduct and Discipline: Fitness to Practice.*

In its most recent version, *Duties of a Doctor*, the booklet on confidentiality was the clearest expressions of the principles of confidentiality. The BMA commissioned Ross Anderson of Cambridge University's Computer Laboratory to use those principles as the base for a data security policy for clinical information, which would enable doctors to fulfil its demands.

There have been similar struggles for statutory regulation of other health care professions, notable dates being the establishment in

1960 of the Council for Professions Supplementary to Medicine (a new act is currently out for consultation);
1983 of the UKCC as the combined registering body for nurses, midwives and health visitors;
1995 the osteopaths' register

Recent international experience has highlighted the need for legal registration of health care professionals and regulation by politically independent disciplinary committees.

Strong, independent medical associations, too, can now be clearly seen as vital not only to protect the individual practitioner against the malicious state, e.g. the 16 year agony of the imprisoned Syrian doctors, but also to protect the human rights of the individual patient, e.g. abuse of psychiatry in the USSR in Stalinist times and the current case in Turkey where doctors have been arrested and will be tried in Adana for failing to give to government the identity of patients who seek treatment after torture (by state agents).

Kennedy identifies the central strand of the traditional doctor-patient relationship that, in general terms, third parties are excluded from the relationship, except in rare and well-defined circumstances. The issue of power is again present, this time in the form of the power of the patient to bind the doctor to keep his secrets and the duty and power of the doctor to respect a promise to do so in the face of a desire of a third party, whether an individual or an institution of the State, to know [1].

Thus Turkish doctors are currently putting their liberty on the line for a principle that in this country doctors are in danger of blindly relinquishing.

And again Kennedy writes: "The obligation of confidence entails that one party has the right to control the dissemination of whatever information she makes available and that the other party to the obligation has no right to disseminate any information, subject to some major reason of public policy. Thus, the key to confidentiality is the right to control access to information as against third parties" [2].

But we are now at a watershed in access to information. Can we preserve medical confidentiality as we move from a world of print to a world of networked computer databases?

Following Caxton's invention in the 15th century, the move from the painstaking perfection of illuminated vellum by monks to the mass production of the printed page opened the doors of learning to secular humanity, standing hungry for knowledge on the steps of the monasteries.

The potential for universal literacy and access to "book knowledge" had been born.

The IT revolution is a culture shift of at least equivalent size to the invention of the printing press, with events on a scale and at a pace and with a potential that are sometimes difficult for professional organisations (and their senior officers) to grasp. The British health care professional organisations are belatedly and painfully recognising that for us knowingly to commit identifiable data to insecure information systems contravenes all tenets of professional good practice. This is not uniquely a problem for medicine and its sister professions. It is a problem for any profession whose clients share identifiable personal information and have a right to believe will be handled confidentially — law, social service, counselling, etc. For doctors, however, recognition of a patients right to privacy is the fundamental of our contract with them.

But as McLean reminds us "Medicine is not simply an exercise of purely clinical skills. It transcends the technical to reach the level of morality by the sharing of respect. Indeed, medicine has long been concerned with questions of ethics, and has long shown a commitment to morality in dealing with the patient — however incomplete ... this ... stems from recognition of the need to view the patient as an autonomous human being, with rights and interests which are identifiable independently of medicine." [3]

"The basic attribute of an effective right of privacy is the individual's ability to control the flow of information concerning or describing him." [4]

In the US health system this has been addressed by General Release Forms

(Consent). On entering a health care facility, the patient is asked to sign a variety of forms. One of these is likely to be an authorization that essentially states that the facility may release medical information concerning the patient to anyone it thinks should have it or to certain named agencies or organizations. Receivers should, however, be liable for an invasion-of-privacy action if they use the medical information for other than the specific purpose for which the health care facility released it to them [5].

Clearly consent under the duress of acute illness is scarcely likely to be considered, and it has been suggested that consent to information sharing should be given in advance of the immediate clinical situation rather like a living will.

IT can give access to information to both health care professions and the public on disease, its processes and progress, pathology and treatment, outcomes and potential for new approaches. Soon every patient with access to a competent teenager will be able to have access to all of this information via Internet.

But medical records held on computer, especially *identifiable* records on large databases, will be equally accessible to those not directly involved in patient care. Accessible to many for whom the patient will not have given consent for access, nor will the patient *know* when their records have been inappropriately accessed. The dangers of large aggregated databases, with poor access control, inadequate data security policies, poorly taught, patchingly implemented with a paucity of monitoring and no legal protection have been demonstrated already in the United States. In America the Privacy Commission recommended that each medical care provider be required to notify an individual on whom it maintains a medical record of the disclosures that may be made of information in the record without the individual's express authorization [6].

The UK medical profession must get its house in order and refuse to use any untried information technology. The first precept of the Hippocratic Oath, or its modern equivalent, the Declaration of Geneva is:

> The health of my patient will be my first concern

Unless technically and legally protected, there will be "information creep" from databases with identifiable patient information potentially being linked to other databases, e.g.

- Social security (justified by the prevention of fraud)
- Home Office (to track and prevent drug abuse / to track illegal immigrants etc)
- Police (justified for the prevention of crime)
- MI5 (recently, and worryingly because of the lack of public accountability, working with the police in prevention and detection of serious crime)

We could categorise these agencies as Big Brother.

As for Big Business —- Big Brother's twin — identifiable data is of equally intense interest; to the insurance companies (life, pension, health), to employment agencies, drug companies (re disease management profiles) and to journalists and politicians — as the source of front page stories or a means of neutering political opponents.

Only last week at BMA House we had a one-day conference on genetic testing of children. That information has the potential to marginalise individuals from infancy, potentially disqualify them from further education (is it worth saving for a college course, one American family asked, if a gene test is positive for late development of a life threatening illness ?) from employment or from insurance, all on the basis perhaps of an identified genetic tendency to develop a disease in mid-life.

Information is power, and here we have the potential for unauthorised access to identifiable personal information effectively crushing the privacy of the doctor/patient relationship between the grindstones of Big Brother and Big Business.

Margaret Thatcher in her first invitation to deliver the Conservative Political Centre lecture in 1968 was much struck as Hugo Young reports in his political biography *One of Us* by the power the government gained through information, and by the looming threat of computerised files of personal data. She waxed uncommonly eloquent on this theme:

> Consider our relations with government departments. We start as a birth certificate; attract a maternity grant; give rise to a tax allowance and possibly a family allowance; receive a national health number when registered with a doctor; receive pension and become a death certificate and death grant, and ... the amount of information collected in the various departments must be fabulous.

She was concerned, in a way she did little to sustain in later years, at the threat this posed to individual privacy. "There would be produced for the first time a personal dossier about each person, on which everything would be recorded. In my view this would place far too much power in the hands of the state over the individual."

Doctors have an ethical duty, I believe, as a profession to ensure that they access competent technical knowledge, expertise and advice in the relevant specialist disciplines to enable the use of IT to enhance the profession's contract with both the individual patient and society).

Were doctors as negligent in their approach to infection control as they are in currently in their approach in information control, then the charge of professional negligence would be seen as eminently reasonable.

Possibly the most internationally influential piece of work from the BMA in the last decade has been *Medicine Betrayed* [8], our report on doctors' involvement in human rights abuses and torture. We energetically, and perhaps cheaply in terms of our own personal comfort, enjoin doctors in totalitarian or pseudo-democratic regimes to put themselves at risk in exposing and refusing to take part in human rights abuses. The British medical profession needs to listen to its own exhortations. To uphold the long traditions of ethical practice we too must act to make real our obligation of confidence. This is a demand on each individual doctor and on each professional organisation.

It was Sir Douglas Black, Chairman of the working party on the participation of doctors in Human Rights Abuses, who suggested the title *Medicine Betrayed.* It is our relationship of trust with the individual patient that British doctors are now on the point of betraying. The lack of both privacy and safety in the handling of medical records stored on insurance company mainframes, has destroyed that trust in the doctor patient relationship in the States. We have been warned: it is on the point of happening here. The lessons laid out so clearly in *Medicine Betrayed* are evident; health care professionals are always the first to see human rights abuses and this include the rights of privacy. A strong independent and resolute national medical association coupled with an independent regulatory body are, surprisingly for some, amongst the strongest defenders of a free society. As Woodward identified in a leader in the BMJ in 1995, medical leadership is essential in this situation [9].

We are involved in trench warfare on a technical battle field with much under cover guerrilla activity. The battle we are fighting is for the continuing existence of independent health care professionals in the UK as against health care technicians. This calls for leadership in the highest order from senior medical figures. They are not asked to risk their freedom, their lives and the possible torture of their families (as are our Turkish colleagues) or but merely to relinquish the comfort of approval in Government circles, future honours and quango placements, (and to risk the embarrassment of being described as Luddite!)

Thus the perspective of medical ethics reveals a political imperative.

Doctors *and* their patients need medical politicians who are ethically driven. As The New Statesman's article of 14 June reminds us,"in the long run politicians who take risks for principle are rewarded".

References

1. Kennedy, I. *Rights and Wrongs in Medicine.* Ed Peter Byrne, Oxford University press (1986)
2. Kennedy, I. *Medicine in Contemporary Society.* Ed Peter Byrne, Oxford University press (1987)
3. McLean, Sheila A. M., *A Patient's Right to Know — Information Disclosure, the Doctor and the Law* Dartmouth Publishing Company Medico-Legal Series (1989)
4. Miller, *Personal Privacy in the Computer Age*, 67 Mich. L. Rev. 1091, 1107 (1968)
5. Annas, George J. *The Rights of Patients: The basic ACLU guide to patients' rights* 2nd ed. Humana Press, Towtowa, New Jersey (1992)
6. Annas, ibid.
7. Young, Hugo *One of Us*, Macmillan, London (1989)
8. British Medical Association, *Medicine Betrayed: The Participation of Doctors in Human Rights Abuses*, Zed Books London 1992
9. Woodward B, *Disclosure and use of personal health information*, BMJ 1996;312:653–4
10. New Statesman, *Shake Rattle and Roll*, 14 June 1996 p 5

Legal Requirements for Computer Security: An American Perspective

David A. Banisar

Electronic Privacy Information Center
666 Pennsylvania Ave, SE, Suite 301
Washington, DC 20003
http://www.epic.org

There are numerous laws in the United States governing the privacy of personal information, including medical records. Many of these laws also mandate that the security of records is also ensured.

The presentation will examine some of the currently existing laws that govern computer security including the Privacy Act of 1974, the Computer Security Act, the Computer Fraud and Abuse Act, federal court decisions, state laws, and international guidelines. It will then examine current proposals for medical privacy bills in the US, including proposals introduced by Senate Bennett, Rep. McDermott, Rep. Condit and the Clinton Heath Security Act.

Finally, the presentation will examine possible model language towards dealing with security issues and some of the technologies that are currently in use such as cryptography, digital signatures, smart cards, and audit trails.

U.S. Health Information Privacy Policy: Theory and Practice

Agneta Breitenstein, J.D.

JRI Health Law Institute
29 Stanhope Street, Boston, MA 02116
(617) 867-7881
e-mail: ag@jri.org

A Marble Monument is erected by the State with an inscription:

The Unknown Citizen

He was found by the Bureau of Statistics to be
One against whom there was no official complaint,
And all the reports of his conduct agree
That in the Modern Sense of an old-fashioned word, he was a saint,
For in everything he did, he served the Greater Community,
Except for the War, till the day he retired,
He worked in a factory and never got fired,
But he satisfied his employers, Fudge Motors, Inc.,
Yet he wasn't a scab or odd in his views,
For his Union reports that he paid all his dues,
(Our report on his Union shows it was sound)
And our Social Psychology workers found
That he was popular with his mates and liked a drink.
The Press are convinced that he bought a paper everyday
And his reactions to advertisements were normal in every way.
Policies taken out in his name prove that he was fully insured,
And his Health-card shows he was once in the hospital, but left it cured.
Both Producers Research and High-Grade Living declare
He was fully sensible to the advantages of the Installment Plan
And had everything necessary to the Modern Man,
A phonograph, a radio, a car, a Frigidaire.
Our researchers into Public Opinion are content
That he held the proper opinions for the time of year;
When there was peace, he was for peace, when there was war, he went.
He was married and added five children to the population,
Which our eugenist says was the right number for a parent of his generation.
And our teachers report that he never interfered with their education.
Was he free? Was he happy? The question is absurd:
Had anything been wrong, we certainly would have heard.

by Anonymous
The New Pocket Anthology of American Verse, Pocket Library 1955

1. Introduction

We are on the threshold of developing the most comprehensive, detailed and powerful database of information that has ever existed. The development of a "womb-to-tomb" computerized medical record promises to remake not only the entire landscape of health care delivery systems, but also to alter fundamentally our notions of human identity in the information age. Within the medical context, some of the most intimate, detailed and potentially devastating bits of information are collected. This information is often collected when we are hurt or sick and vulnerable to those people whom we entrust with our care during a crisis. The information thus rendered sheds light on aspects of ourselves that in nearly every other context we might otherwise keep to ourselves.

Upon promises that computerized information systems will speed information to doctors in emergency rooms and allow world class surgeons to operate on patients thousands of miles away, we are rushing headlong toward placing our comprehensive medical records into a computerized environment. And although there has been a host of grandiose suggestions about the benefits of such a system, we are as yet unclear about the benefits which will accrue in any but the most dire or extreme of situations. What *is* becoming increasingly clear, however, is that computerized health information systems and technology pose enormous challenges and risks to the confidentiality of health information and the autonomy of patients in choosing modalities of health care.

Computers and privacy are not by definition antithetical. Computers present new challenges that test the bounds of established privacy policy and law. The greatest challenge of computerized medical records is not the technical security of such information. Technology is limitless in its ability to make unauthorized access to information nearly impossible. The greater challenge is to define who will be admitted to the realm of authorized users or specifically to define the parameters of confidentiality in light of the fundamental change brought about in the nature and quality of information within a computerized context. In the information age, invention is the true mother of necessity. Computerized record systems make data infinitely accessible and usable. And because computers can do incredible things with information, many adopt a mentality which dictates that suddenly all those things that were not necessary when they were impossible suddenly become essential. Technology *has* allowed us to create databases capable of answering our queries and manipulating information in ways that a few years ago would have been possible or required an army of file clerks. Technology *will* allow for interactive "bedside" assistants that will recommend treatment modalities and assist, or, in some cases even replace doctors. As a result, we suddenly need all of the new information and assistance that can be generated by this technology. Unless, however, we develop strong, definable confidentiality policies, we will not be able to determine who should legitimately use and/or gain access to all of the new information. Phrased alternatively, if we throw open the doors of access to anyone who knocks then our technical ability to secure information will be meaningless.

In this paper, I will attempt to describe the current debate occurring in the U.S. in the policy arena with respect to medical privacy. I will focus on the contours of the conflict between an individual's right to medical privacy and those who claim a need to access and use personally identifiable medical information. I will also attempt to suggest some concrete policy principles designed to negotiate this conflict. Finally, I hope to illustrate that the American public and ultimately the international community have critical decisions to make about who will and will not have access to personally identifiable medical information without our consent and how technology will be used in this regard. Ultimately, we may decide, in some circumstances, to allow some access to our health information. In most, however, we may and should decide that the ultimate cost to our health and our health care system will be greater than the short term gain to be won through unrestrained access to identifiable medical data. In any case, individuals must be given specific, legislative tools useful in maintaining control of personal data as it enters vast information systems. In making privacy policy decisions, we must proceed carefully and think creatively about ways in which the various interests at stake may be balanced. In many cases, I believe that just as technology has been the tool used to create many of the problems we face, technology will also likely help us to solve some of the most challenging questions in this arena.

2. The problem described

When we were young, we used to think that if a friend told us a secret which we then told another friend, it would be acceptable as long as we made our second friend promise not to tell anyone else. Inevitably our second friend would go on, however, to repeat our original breach by telling yet another friend, again, in exchange for the promise that they too would tell no one else. As we all know from our childhood experiences with secrecy, this always led to the demise of the original confidence. Our secret would get around to everyone on our playground, inevitably fueled by the mere fact that it was a secret and it's telling an act of trust between intimates.

This childhood example accurately describes the mistaken and disturbing shift currently occurring in the U.S. debate about the confidentiality of health information.[1] Massive centralized databases of computerized medical records are seen as an inevitability. The circle of those who claim to have a "need-to-know" is ever widening. None of our previous experience with confidentiality has prepared us for the distinctly new challenges posed by the computer. As a result, the dialogue is being shifted away from a consent driven model of confidentiality and toward a threat model of security where the paramount concern is protecting against the outside hacker or other obviously unauthorized user .[2] In other words, promises of "security" are being substituted for the original promise of "confidentiality" essential to the successful medical relationship. What remains less well examined, therefore, is the threat posed to medical confidentiality and medical care by the fact that an increasing number of people and entities are demanding and getting, via the computer, access to sensitive information and patients are increasingly less able to refuse these intrusions for fear if losing health benefits, employment, etc.. We have seen this already in the conflicts that have arisen over the Clipper chip and key escrow. We can have state-of-the-art encryption and privacy tools, but someone is always going to demand access. The question is how can we *restore the confidence* in confidential medical communications and reduce the coercive influences that now prevent us from ever truly exercising voluntary consent. Ultimately, I would submit, that we must think carefully about the amount and type of information that we entrust to computerized systems regardless of how secure the system will be against unauthorized intrusion. As I hope to highlight at the end of this paper, I believe our ability to control our identities may be at stake.

3. Overview of the current debate in the U.S.

3.1 The ethical dilemma

The medical profession has always struggled with balancing the autonomy of patients with the desire to make them healthy despite themselves. This experience is shared by many, including my own legal profession. As professionals, we study and practice for a lifetime in order to know what is the best course of action for our clients or patients. Those we serve often come with great need or in times of dire crisis. The desire to take control of the situation and ultimately of the patient is often strong. And when patients refuse to heed the best advice or choose not to elect what we believe is the best course of treatment or action, we are frustrated in the very purpose we have chosen to serve with our lives.

With respect to computerized medical records systems, many view the prospect of instant access to detailed medical records through digital systems to be a great clinical tool for the treatment of patients. Indeed, in a variety of contexts this will be true. What remains less clear, however, is the ethical impact of creating a computerized health information system that makes it impossible for clinicians to treat patients unless their health information is computerized.

While record keeping has historically remained within the control of health care professionals, the exigencies of the current health care system demand that health care professionals surrender tight control of this information to health insurers, employers, computer professionals and information management entities. The relationship between doctors and medical records is becoming more protracted. Increasingly, health information technology companies are seeking to put computerized platforms for the collection of health information directly at the point of care.[3] By placing the computer next to the patient's bedside, as it were, with a pipeline leading directly to a massive database which is accessible to the health insurers or other entities, doctors are losing the ability to have one-on-one relationships with patients. There is another actor in the exam room. Ethically speaking, as doctors become unable to practice without the aid of such computers, they can no longer represent that there is any sort of confidential relationship unless the patient knows who has access to the computerized information.

Similarly, increasing reliance on the computer as a diagnostic and treatment tool is beginning to encroach upon the very methodology of health care. With wholesale collection and standardization of health information into "code sets" (standard terminological or numerical codes representing clinical information traditionally presented in narrative form), we are paving the way for development of complex medical "algorithms" which would be used at the point of care to augment or even supplant the physician's role as a professional. This event was presaged by the developing use of "diagnosis-related groups"(DRGs) and other quantitative code sets by the government, insurers and HMOs to guide decision making in the treatment and utilization review (UR) process. Increasingly, "case managers" are using DRGs and other algorithms to evaluate clinical treatment decisions *before* care is ever administered and based solely on the analysis of DRGs gleaned from health information collected and stored in a computer. Such a process has been touted as "cost-containment." What seems to have escaped notice in this scenario, is the effect this has on the practice of medicine as all treatment decisions become subject to the formulaic response of payers as they accept or reject the claims made by doctors trying to treat patients. The medical record is becoming less of a tool for clinicians to memorialize and plan treatment and becoming more of the tool of the payor in controlling the practice of medicine. The translation of clinical information into DRGs and code sets is indicative of this shift.

It is particularly worth noting here that by placing computers at each bedside, health information technology companies are also explicitly seeking "ownership" of the information collected.[4] For health care professionals, this would be a profound shift away from the traditional understanding of medical records as an aide in the clinical process. We must remind ourselves, that clinicians are ethically and legally responsible for the way in which health care is delivered. Such a profound change in the methodology of health care must be addressed by clinicians.

3.2 Information in the age of shifting resource allocation

The current debate concerning health information confidentiality must be understood in the context of the increasingly desperate and unresolved debate about health care resource allocation in the U.S.. The high cost and unavailability of health care resources in the U.S. threaten the viability of the current health care system. We have recognized as a nation that we are spending a tremendous amount of our national resources on health care expenses. As a result, efforts toward cost cutting, risk management and managed care have caused great shifts in the way in which health care is delivered. These shifts have caused movement away from fee-for-service payment of medical professionals and toward managed care systems that bind the provider and payer interests together. We are rapidly moving away from a singular patient/consumer-doctor/provider decision making model and toward a resource allocative model, where the patient, though consumer, has the least leverage in controlling the amount and type of resources consumed.

On a large scale we can see this by the rapid rise of capitated systems and health maintenance organizations (HMO). The capitated model works on the theory that if provider and payer interests are fused, the provider will be incentivized toward suppressing costs. In this system, an individual life is capitated. The money is fronted for the life by the entity paying the premium (the employer in most circumstances), and the provider delivers and plans care, keeping the difference between the amount paid and the cost of care provided. In this model, the provider bears the risk and is therefore incentivized toward keeping care costs low. This simplified description differs from the old fee-for-service system in that the interests of the payer and the provider are fused and the patient is at least once removed from the equation. In capitated systems, the decision making process regarding the type and quantity of care is heavily weighted by the economic interest of the provider/payer.

The shift toward binding the provider and payer profoundly effects the developing models for resource allocation in both the public and private spheres. We see this in both the ability of patients to access and refuse certain care. Allocative models, such as that described by Michael Rie[5], have attempted to balance the finite resources of available in the public realm with the needs of those who have no way to pay for health care themselves. The model known as "the Oregonian ICU" describes a "moral" system for rationing care in cases where intensive health care resources are limited. This model presumes that in those cases where the patient's "prognostic score" indicates that the chances of survival are low, no care, other than palliative treatment will be administered. While, on the one hand, such a model bespeaks the probable and regrettable reality of our current system, it fails to recognize that whereas once doctors, patients and families made decisions, the public interest in conserving limited resources will increasingly trump individual decision making based upon quantitative analysis. Quantitative analysis in this realm relies upon the ability of computers to generate the data necessary for outcome determination.

Privatized systems are beginning to reflect this same trend away from individualized decision making. Many employers have begun to impose certain health regimens upon employees under threat of termination or fine in an effort to lower health costs prospectively.[6] Employees are losing the ability to make their own decisions about their dietary, exercise or other habits with a health impact because the employer, in many cases, is paying for the consequences. As with public rationing systems, control of decision making with respect to health care is being gradually taken away from patients and handed over to private and public care managers. Patients are losing the ability to make independent decisions about the amount and type of care the consume or decline.

3.3 Health information as a health management tool

In this context, information has become an essential part of the cost management equation. Comprehensive computerized health records are seen as the key that will unlock the door to significant cost savings and care management.[7] In 1991, the Institute of Medicine (IOM) called the computer based patient record an "essential technology" reasoning that the computerization of the medical record will allow for the easy collection and collation of the cradle-to-grave medical record which would then be made accessible to other health care providers, researchers, cost managers, payers, regulators and policy makers. The IOM report entitled, *The Computer-Based Patient Record: An Essential Technology For Health Care*[8], states quite clearly that such a tool is invaluable for the development of an integrated health care system. Integration in this context refers, not only to integrated care models, but also integration of care and payer systems.

Based on the notion that the computer will allow instant access to the comprehensive medical record, the report identifies at least two tiers of uses that would be greatly facilitated. Among the first tier uses are health care providers, patients, care support staff, and risk managers. But also included among these first tier of uses are billing and reimbursement[9]. In this model, as with the HMO model, the provider and payer are similarly situated with respect to access to the computerized record. This suggestion is a radical departure from any historic notion of the primary use of the patient record. Allowing full computerized access to the medical record by the payer can only be justified by the notion that the payer should be allowed to review the minutiae of all care decisions made by providers—in essence, to practice by proxy. By this I mean, that by giving the payer the complete record, we are validating the notion that, for any given treatment for which a provider has billed, a payer will be given the opportunity to ratify or reject such a decision based on the information gleaned from the medical record.

3.4 The legislative response

Shortly after the IOM report, Bill Clinton launched his campaign for the "National Health Security Act." Contained within this proposal was a plan for the creation of a national health care database.[10] This database was intended to embody the recommendations made in the IOM report and serve as the informational backbone of the proposed health care system. The proposal mandated the standardization of all health care data and the computerization of all medical encounters within the national database. All of the information would have been managed under a unique identifier, likely to be the social security number. This system was viewed as the primary cost containment monitoring system that would be used in deploying health resources and the monitoring costs as judged against the global health care budget. The Clinton health care plan stated that the network would support "analytic needs, such as monitoring budgets, measuring access, and state accountability, assessing quality, among states, health plans, health alliances and the federal government."[11] In contrast to the chaos which characterizes the current health care system, this centralized information system seemed entirely efficient. In terms of confidentiality, however, such a system was a disaster. This database would have led to the creation of the single largest, most comprehensive source of the most intimate details of every American's life. Its impact is difficult to assess in anything other than the most hyperbolic terms.

The Clinton plan has died. The notion of computerizing and standardizing patient data lives on. The model has been renamed "Administrative Simplification[12]" in its most recent legislative incarnations and was just passed over the fierce objection of privacy advocates nationwide. Administrative Simplification works much like the federal standardization of railroad track width in the last century. While Administraive Simplification does not mandate the massive computerization of medical records, it makes such a system technically possible by doing two things. First, it requires that every individual be assigned a unique identifier, thus allowing every patient to be tracked throughout the health care system. Second, it establishes a standard computerized medical language to be applied to the entire medical record—a computerized health data "Esperanto" if you will—which will enable all of the various public and private data systems to speak to one another . This legislation is truly elegant because it is not so much a mandate which creates the database as a systematic "greasing" of the wheels of electronic health data systems. It does not legislate the creation of a government run database, but instead provides the necessary elements that will allow private companies to develop and link massive medical record data repositories. It will not matter where any specific electronic medical record lies within this data system. The nature of electronic media within the framework of this system will allow anyone with access to the system to assemble all of the medical records or other health data related to any individual almost instantaneously. Most frighteningly, the majority of this data will be held and controlled by large private data companies who count medical records as corporate assets and claim ownership of the data even if they never got consent to hold or use this information at any point. This provision was passed without any requirement that the patient consent to the computerization of their data. It is clear, it seems, that if technology such as this, which promises such sweeping effects, is implemented without patient consent or even over the objections of the patient, its primary function is to serve the health care system rather than the patients.

3.5 The Bennett bill - S. 1360

In the context of the nascent national database, Senator Robert Bennett of Utah introduced the Medical Records Confidentiality Act of 1995 (S.1360). S.1360 has been touted as a "patient's rights bill" requiring consent for disclosure of health information. It is clear, however, upon closer inspection that S. 1360 suffers the same fundamental problems as the national database, in that its primary goal is to facilitate the massive computerization of medical records without consent.

Senator Bennett, when introducing the bill, stated that its primary goal was to override the various state laws impeding the development of national and regional databases of medical information[13]. He was referring to the fact that while there exists no federal right of privacy with respect to medical records, nearly every state in the union has enacted some sort of privacy law protecting medical records. Each, however, is different in its scope and interpretation. S.1360 has looked to some as though it would be a net gain for privacy in so far as it established a generalizable rule requiring consent for disclosures of medical records. What it gave on the one hand, however, it quickly took away with the other. S.1360 has, in all its various forms (it has been redrafted several times throughout the debate), consistently held three things: 1) state law will be preempted with respect to medical privacy paving the way for uninhibited interstate transfer of computerized medical data; 2) computerization of medical information can occur without patient consent; and 3) independent computerized information managers will be allowed to stand in the shoes of health care providers when it comes to the holding and management of medical information. These three things, coupled with the fact that all of the entities that claim a "need to know", including law enforcement, public health , research, accreditation bodies, and health information management agencies, are given access without consent, meant that S.1360 promises little in return for what it gave away. There is nothing in S. 1360 that would remedy the potentially devastating effects of the national health care database.

4. Essential elements of medical privacy policy

S. 1360 garnered support initially because, when judged against individual state statutes, standards and practices governing paper medical records, S.1360 seemed to be appropriately protective. In light of both the rapid changes occurring in health information technology and in the commodification of health care, this bill fell well short of its articulated goals. The old standards of informed consent must be adapted to fit the new challenges posed by computerized medical data and the ever growing involvement of payers and other entities in the treatment process. The choice of whether or not computerize records and decisions regarding who will have access to such records run far ahead of the traditional notion of consent. Consent is neither a protection nor a barrier when both payers and providers occupy a far superior bargaining position in relation to patients such that patients must consent or lose coverage. Addressing this challenge is fundamental to any true notion of medical confidentiality.

There are four key elements to an effective medical privacy policy: notice; informed, non-coerced consent; limited insider access; and non-consensual disclosure allowed only in specified and compelling circumstances. Each element must be evaluated in the context of computerized informational abilities. For purposes of focus and brevity, this paper will discuss the first two of these elements, notice and informed, non-coerced consent.

4.1 Notice

More than any other single factor, notice is absolutely essential to the proper protection of medical confidentiality. Regardless of what rights individuals are given to control personal information, they will be difficult, if not entirely impossible to exercise if patients have no notice of who has their medical information and why. Effective notice requires that any individual whose health information is held by another should have clear and unambiguous information regarding: who has that information, what is the nature of the information held by that entity, where and how is that information stored, and why does this entity want or have access to this data.

Notice:

Active

Disclosure and Use Specified

Use of Agents Specified

Inspection, Copying, and Correction Allowed

Currently, most people in the U.S. have no idea of who "owns" or has access to the bulk of their personal information. This is most clearly demonstrated in the field of credit reporting. Credit reporting in the U.S. is a large and crucial business. Credit reports are routinely required by banks, landlords, employers, insurers, creditors, etc.. The weight of one's credit report is difficult to quantify. Yet, despite its pivotal role in the lives of most Americans, most are ignorant of the whereabouts, contents, owners and uses of these reports. Owing to the fact that most people have no notice about who has their credit report, this information is traded freely on the open market with little or no limitation. In the U.S., one's credit history is virtually a public record. Without adequate notice provisions, health information will move into a similarly mysterious and ethereal realm, away from the bright lights of necessary public scrutiny.

Notice is the first, small, but crucial step toward restoring control of personal health information. Notice must be active. Anyone who holds health information must notify the patient that they have such data. Anyone who is sending health information must notify the patient of the intended recipient within the context of the consent process. Resistance to notice stems in part from industry fear that a transparent information system will cause consumer disgust. This is certainly a well founded fear. Others have voiced objections to this principle on the grounds that it would be administratively burdensome to require an affirmative obligation of notice. And while there is no dispute that notice will require additional expense and effort, it is clear that patients should not be alone in bearing the burden that industrial secrecy places upon them. Phrased alternatively, information management companies should not be the only ones left with any privacy.

This subject of notice becomes particularly complex in the context of the rapid commodification of health care. In days past, we confided in our doctors who, under the Hippocratic Oath, were bound to protect our confidences. Generally speaking, doctors used to be independent professionals who used medical records as *aide-mémoire* and little else. As noted above, however, health care is becoming a business with a bottom line. Services are segmented, outsourced, corporatized and subcontracted. Doctors are becoming but a small cog in an ever growing machine. A health care "entity" such as a hospital may in fact comprise many independently contracted service providers. Similarly, tasks once within the province and control of licensed health care professionals have been subcontracted to entities outside the traditional health care realm. Information and computer services are a clear example. Medical records are seldom managed "within" the same organization that delivers care. Medical records services have proliferated and promise to grow exponentially as computer technology makes the management of information increasingly complex and geographically fluid.

This fact poses a grave problem for confidentiality. As a matter of policy, no one should be able to hide within the various corporate veils which are gradually wrapping themselves around the health care system. Health information is imparted to doctors by patients within a health care model which legally requires consent. Disclosure of information to agents who are standing in the shoes of the provider and using the doctor's visage, as it were, is directly in conflict with the concept of consent. If one uses an independent contractor for the managing health information, notice of such usage and consent must implemented.

Coupled with active notice, any entity that possesses medical records must allow the subject of the information the opportunity and functional ability to access, inspect, copy and correct such information. The increasing reliance on health information by insurers, employers, educators and the government requires that patients have the right and real ability to monitor and correct the information. Many health care professionals, especially within the mental health profession, resist open access to the record by patients. It is imperative to note, however, that health information is moving further and further out of the strict control of health care professionals. Because clinicians cannot protect the absolute confidentiality of their records, patients have an ever increasing need and commensurate right to inspect and correct this data.

Some clinicians and privacy advocates have proposed that, especially in the mental health context, clinicians be allowed to keep "personal notes" separate from the record. These personal notes would not be defined by content but rather by the fact that they would never be released to anyone under any circumstances. Such an exception is promising from the strict perspective of medical privacy. At the point at which such notes are released to anyone, however, equity demands that the patient must have the absolute right to inspect and correct such information. This policy can be expanded to other medical professions. It should not, and cannot functionally be expanded outside the clinical realm. The judgment to restrict access to such notes must only be based upon a clinician's determination that the information would jeopardize the health or safety of the individual. Non-medical personnel cannot make such a judgment.

4.2 Informed, non-coerced consent

The principle of consent is central to patient centered privacy policy. Indeed the concept of informed consent grows out of the health care profession as a whole. Legally, medical treatment delivered without consent is actionable as battery. Ethically, consent is essential to the autonomy of the individual. With respect to health information, it is most helpful to imagine that medical records are an extension of the physical body of the patient. Just as a doctor would not operate (except in extraordinary circumstances) on a patient's leg without consent, so to would such a doctor be prohibited from using or disclosing health information without securing authorization from the subject of such information.

4.2.1 Access to health data must be limited for employers, insurers or schools

Voluntary consent is difficult to exercise fully in the American medical system because consent is generally coerced. Health information is required by insurers for payment of health claims. Failure to consent generally results in a denial of the claim. Similarly coercive situations exist where employers and schools demand medical information in return for employment and education. Because these entities have superior bargaining power with respect to the patient, there is no opportunity to exercise truly voluntary consent.

This fact poses a significant problem with respect to privacy policy in the current health care context. Without the ability to make a truly voluntary decision in most of the instances where medical information is disclosed, it is questionable whether we can truly call coerced authorization for disclosure consent at all. As a result, it is absolutely critical that the ability of insurers, employers, schools and other entities to coerce consent from patients be curtailed.

In approaching this problem, we must first consider the assumptions traditionally made justifying access by insurers, employers or schools. These entities have a commercial rather than a clinical interest in the information contained in these records. As such they should be separately regulated as "commercial users" of medical records. Commercial users are distinct from doctors and other health care providers treating patients. The direct provision of health care is the traditional "clinical use" for health data. Health care providers and facilities in this context should be regulated as "clinical users." Making this distinction as a definitional matter is essential to the adequate medical privacy policy. Once the distinction is made, the clinical context can be insulated from plenary access by commercial users. The flow of information from the clinical realm to the commercial realm can be regulated, restoring the ability of patients to prevent coerced consent. Rights granted within this context must be common to all patients. Only by establishing a community standard which makes the privacy of medical data common to all patients can any single individual resist the demands of the commercial realm.

In those instances where access can be justified, information must remain protected within the given environment in which it is located. For the purposes of this paper, I will discuss certain mechanism which may be used in the insurance context, since that is the arena in which this question most frequently comes up.

Insurance has long justified its access to health data on the premise that such information is necessary to review and authorize payment for treatment. The amount and type of data necessary have increased as the involvement of the insurance entities in the delivery of health care has expanded (see discussion above). In any event, detailed health data should not travel to the insurance company. Generally insurance entities should have access to basic administrative billing information such as date of service, treatment, diagnosis and complexity of service. Beyond that, however, only independent peer reviewers of the same or higher professional credentials as the clinician whose treatment is being reviewed should have access to the detailed records for purposes of quality assurance or utilization review. This portion of the medical record should be provided to the reviewer with the patient's name or other identifying information removed and replaced by a policy number or other appropriate identifier. The decision of this reviewer should be reported to the insurance entity under this identifier. The detailed record should then remain only accessible to the reviewer. In this way, the detailed record and the patient's name and other identifying information would remain separate from each other, thus preserving the confidentiality of the patient. Similarly, only a licensed health care professional would review the very detailed record. This preserves the clinical nature of the treatment record and decision making process.

Informed,

Non-Coerced Consent:

Access by Insurers, Employers or Schools Limited

Protection Must Follow the Information

Collection of Data Minimized

Computerization not Required

Longitudinal Records not Required

4.2.2 Protection must follow the information

Typically medical confidentiality laws have been drawn around the professional relationship between doctors and patients. As a result, once the medical record leaves the doctor's office, the protection is also lost. This was not a concern in days past where medical records rarely, if ever left the clinical context. But because people other than health care professionals are increasingly accessing medical records, the requirement of consent must extend beyond the traditional medical context. This can be done by having the consent requirement attach to the information by definition. By attaching the requirement of consent to the information itself, a policy can assure that the patient will retain control even when the information must flow. With such a requirement, consent must be secured with each new use or disclosure, regardless who holds or uses such information. This principle is especially important as health information is used more frequently by all of the non-clinical entities that are increasingly interested in the records. From an equitable perspective, this principle makes sense. Protections which previously attached as part of the professional obligations of doctors are out of date because health information is not restricted to the health profession.

4.2.3 Only the minimal information necessary should be used or disclosed

At one time, the aggregation of health information was administratively very burdensome. Paper based medical records could only accumulate in vast and largely inaccessible libraries of inert information. With computerization, however, vast computerized warehouses of information where data can be quickly analyzed, searched, cross-referenced and indexed are not only possible but growing. In this context, it is essential that only the most limited amount of information be disclosed in any circumstance.

This precept promises to remake a good deal of traditional medical practice. Doctors have always had the luxury of collecting family and health histories from patients as a routine part of health care. Patients volunteer this information because they trust their doctors to know what they need. Patients assume that doctors need information to treat them properly. Increasingly, however, quality assurance and cost containment interests are pushing doctors to collect data which is extraneous to the particular medical encounter at hand, but which furthers the aims of the insurer as they attempt to control costs and predict potential exposure. In this regard, the trusting relationship between doctors and patients is being exploited by other entities wishing to know, for instance, whether a patient wears a bike helmet or a seat belt. This information might be sought by a doctor who is performing a routine check-up because the payer network to which s/he belongs has mandated that their physicians collect such data.

This type of informational "trawlling" can only be curtailed if doctors refrain from collecting and/or using only the information that is justifiable for clinical treatment. This principle is especially true in the genetic context, where the collection of data, as a threshold issue, can be the most damaging. Family health history can be a very strong indicator of genetic predisposition. And though there may be some clinical benefits by collecting and analyzing such data, patients must be aware that such data may hurt their ability to obtain or retain insurance if a genetic predisposition is detected. Doctors have an ethical responsibility to notify and counsel patients on the amount and type of information that will be collected within the doctor/patient relationship.

4.2.4 Patients must have option not to computerize information

This principle is central to the protection of privacy in the information age. Typically people disagree with this concept because they misunderstand the profound implications of computerized records.

The ability to decline to computerize is central because computerized medical records are fundamentally different from paper. Computerized records are not simply an alternative method for the storage and retrieval of information. A fully computerized patient record will allow commercial users to alter significantly the decision making process of doctors and nurses at the point of care. Similarly, data stored digitally can be manipulated, matched, analyzed and stored infinitely. The health information technology industry refers to the fully computerized health information system as "decision support service[14]" not a "storage and retrieval service." In this model, as described above, a computer terminal will be sitting at the bedside of the patient with the comprehensive record available to the doctor. In addition, the payer, the cost containment manager, utilization reviewer, the risk manager or even an "expert system" designed to offer recommendations at any given point in the delivery of health care will be able to participate in "real-time" offering "decisional support" to the treating health care professional. These actors will be in the room participating in the health care delivery process without the knowledge and consent of the patient. Without the ability to decline to have our medical records computerized we, as patients, will lose the ability to choose who will be practicing medicine on our bodies.

The extent of this problem was recently demonstrated in a case recently settled in Minnesota in October of 1995[15]. In this case, the attorney general of that state sued Merck Pharmaceuticals for consumer protection violations. Merck owns a subsidiary called Medco, an administrator of a drug benefit plan used by the majority of insurers in the region. As a routine practice Merck was reviewing the records of patients served by Medco. When Merck found doctors prescribing medications produced by another pharmaceutical company, Merck would contact the doctors and attempt to convince them to switch the prescription to a Merck product. Such contacts were little more than direct marketing based upon the confidential records of the patients. If we create a computerized platform that offers real-time "decision support service", we risk seriously corrupting the independent clinical judgment of health care professionals. Despite any clinical benefits which maybe offered by such a system, patients retain the right to decline to be treated by such a mechanism. Returning to our earlier analogy, it is illegal and unethical for a doctor to tell a patient that they must either submit themselves to a particular treatment modality or go untreated, when a perfectly reasonable alternative modality is available. It would be entirely unethical to create a comprehensive computerized information system and then force every patient to submit their information and ultimately their care to such a system without their consent. Without the ability to decline computerization patients and doctors risk becoming part of a vast health care algorithm which is executed via the Internet.

4.2.5 Longitudinal records should not be created except by the patient

Limiting the creation of longitudinal records flows directly from the principle requiring consent for computerization. Information increases in power exponentially as it is aggregated. In a computerized system, it is possible to identify individuals based upon the inferential matching of a few bits of data. The more data are contained in a system, the more easily a match can be made. The aggregation of disparate medical records into a comprehensive longitudinal record threatens the ability of any person to remain anonymous in any circumstance where privacy or anonymity are essential. For instance, if a patient were to volunteer for a research project regarding breast cancer and the subsequent publication of the research included a brief abstract of this patient's history with identifiable information removed, it would be possible for anyone with access to a computerized medical database to match the "unidentified" data to this patient's identified record by matching the few abstract details to the comprehensive record. This would then eliminate the ability of patients to participate safely in research, get anonymous HIV testing, drug or alcohol counseling, abortions etc., or in any project where any few bits data about them might be available.

In those circumstances where patients may *desire* to computerize a longitudinal record, having been adequately warned of the described above hazards, systems should be designed to segregate information within a networked system using a key system or encryption to prevent the pooling of data within a single access level. Computerized systems can be designed to segregate access at a variety of levels, thus creating "virtual segregation" even if all of the data are linked or stored within a single server.

Any effort to control the development of longitudinal records in the U.S. must take into account the impact that the standard code sets and the unique health identifiers, mandated by Administrative Simplification (see discussion above). will have on the ability of patients to control computerized data. Administrative simplification eliminates the need for an independently constructed computerized architecture for health data. The Internet will provide sufficient capability to make every health data repository accessible. Given the technical *fait accompli* which we now face, it is absolutely critical that patients remain able to prevent the wide area accessibility now made possible. This is where previous notions of privacy fail entirely. Physical barriers have historically made the collection of longitudinal records a matter of collecting paper from various sources. In a digital system, there are no physical barriers. Indeed, physicality itself is eliminated. Patient consent must, therefore, be obtained in any instance where data is to be classified under a unique identifier or to be aggregated from disparate sources. Functionally a patient must be able to obtain health care without surrendering their unique identifier, especially if they are self-paying for care. Requiring the unique identifier and/or the computerization of medical data as a condition of accessing health care is tantamount to shoving a patient into a machine from which they cannot escape.

5. Conclusion

In days past, individual identity was defined by our presence and reputation in a community or a market place. These areas were physical locations where communication was limited. In the digital era which has since dawned, physical space has been compressed into non-existence. Similarly data about an individual can be collected, stored and made accessible by anyone. Increasingly, as we have seen with credit reports, decisions are being made about us based upon the data collected *about* us but not *from* us. Our identities then have come within the control of those control the means by which these data are created and made accessible. To the extent that medical data contains some of the most intimate details of our existence, the necessity for controlling this data is essential to controlling the our new identity in the digital age. Medical privacy policy must facilitate the ability of individuals to control, at any moment, the amount, type and quality of data about them as it resides in computerized systems. As Mark Dery has noted in his book, Escape Velocity: Cyberculture at the End of the Twentieth Century[16], the computer promises to reverse the biblical prophecy from John, "the word made flesh" and remake it into "the flesh made word" or in this case binary code. Such a radical transformation cannot happen surreptitiously and under the benevolent guise of medical care. Its effects will be too profound.

6. Notes

1 I will use the term "health information" in place of "medical record" throughout this paper. Definitionally speaking, I am referring to all information collected by an individual which relates to their physical, mental state, care, treatment or payment for such treatment. I am attempting to broadly define this information beyond that traditionally known within the context of the notes taken or created by a doctor/nurse and contained in a paper file in a medical office. We will look more closely at the implications of this definition later in the paper.

2 The author was recently invited to address a committee at the National Academy of Sciences analyzing security in computerized patient records. The committee stated at the outset of the discussion that its task was to analyze the security of patient records in terms of a "threat model." Threats were defined as those things which might "breach" the security systems designed to protect medical records. It was clear from the discussion which ensued that the committee had completely neglected to address the more real threats posed to confidentiality by those who would be granted permission to access computerized medical records. The paradigm was shifted away from threats to medical confidentiality and toward threats to computerized medical records security.

3 Alex Brown & Sons, Inc. *Health Information Technology Industry Overview*, Oct. 13, 1995; p.13.

4 Id.

5 *The Oregonian ICU: Multi-Tiered Monetarized Morality in Health Insurance Law*, Journal of Law Medicine & Ethics, 23 (1995): 149-66.

6 See Christine Gorman, *Big Brother Wants You Healthy*, Time, 62: May 6, 1996. This article describes various schemes imposed by employers where employees may be fired or fined if they engage in certain behaviors such as smoking or failing to wear seat belts.

7 See Lawrence O. Gostin, *Health Information Privacy*, Cornell Law Review, Spring, 1995

8 Richard S. Dick and Elaine B. Steen, eds. (Washington, D.C., National Academy Press, 1991)

9 U.S. Congress, Office of Technological Assessment, Protecting Privacy of Computerized Medical Information: Washington, D.C., U.S. Government Printing Office: 1993 Sep., No.: OTA-TCT-576, p. 23. Diagram created by the American Health Information Management Association based upon information taken from IOM report *The Computer-Based Patient Record: An Essential Technology For Health Care.*

10 The White House Domestic Policy Council, The President's Health Security Plan; 123, (Times Books, 1993)

11 Id. at 128.

12 Public Law: 104-191, Subtitle F, Part C.

13 Statements on Introduced Bills and Joint Resolutions, Senate October 24, 1995; Statement of Senator Robert Bennett, 2nd Session, 104th Congress; S. Rep. No.____

14 Alex Brown, Inc. at 21.

15 PRNewswire, October 25, 1995; *Minnesota Takes the Lead On Agreement to Protect 41 Million Americans*; at 1.

16 Grove Press, Emeryville, California, 1996

Managing Health Data Privacy and Security: A Case Study from New Zealand

Roderick Neame, MA,PhD,MB,Bchir

Health Information Consulting,
Homestall House, Homestall Lane,
Faversham, Kent ME13 8UT, England
Email 100764.3727@Compuserve.com
http://www.health-info.co.uk

Abstract

The past decade has seen a rapid upsurge of interest and concern relating to protecting the privacy of personal information. Some countries have enacted adequate privacy legislation: others have not. Protection of personal information privacy is generally accepted as a fundamental civil right: failure to respect this right is widely seen as associated more with oppressive and totalitarian regimes than with free democracies.

Nowhere is the issue brought into clearer focus than in the context of wide area health information systems. Patients expect the information they share with their clinician in the context of receiving care to be respected and kept confidential, whether or not that data is seen by others as potentially sensitive. Providers of care services expect to be able to do this, but are increasingly finding that administrators, and especially purchasers of care services, are requiring access to information which is inconsistent with this ethic.

Introduction of computer systems offers improved accessibility and mobility of data, bringing clear benefits, but also risks, especially to confidentiality. The popular perception, based on past experiences, is that such systems do not protect personal privacy: where security is suspect, information will be withheld and the usefulness of the system will be degraded. Systems where privacy and security issues are inadequately managed will never be able to fulfill their intended purpose, and therefore represent poor value for the money that must be invested in them.

This paper addresses some of the key issues, and outlines how they have been successfully addressed in the context of a national health information system in New Zealand.

Introduction

Most patients expect that the information they give to their doctor in the context of receiving proper medical attention will be treated as confidential. The Hippocratic Oath, which guides doctors' ethicalbehaviour, includes the statement:

> *"Whatever in connection with my professional practice, or not in connection with it, I see or hear, in the life of men, which ought not to be spoken of abroad, I will not divulge, as reckoning that all such should be kept secret."*

Health records stored on paper are perversely secure because of the intrinsic difficulty of accessing and searching them, and this hinders their usefulness both to users and to abusers who might breach their confidentiality. However where records are stored in computerised information management systems, they become more accessible so creating the potential for wider and more systematic abuse of personal privacy: this is further increased as systems are linked into regional, national and global health networks. Public and practitioner concern over health information confidentiality is growing in the context of a data protection environment that is often perceived as inadequate, ineffective and lagging behind public expectations.

The role of the patient medical record has changed. In the past the record was primarily for the information of the care provider, to act as a clinical aide-mémoire and, where appropriate, as an archival record of care. Now, however, elements of patient records must be shared widely between professionals to support the activities of care teams, but they must also be shared with non-medical staff to support the needs of business, fiscal and contract management, as well as for quality assurance, research and other purposes. The list of 'authorised' users of the record is increasing, inevitably putting pressure on existing mechanisms and conventions regarding protection of personal privacy.

Medical records contain a wealth of information, some elements of which may be of significant commercial value. Consideration of the possible exploitation of medical records for profit leads into the issue of ownership of the records themselves. There is general agreement at the societal level, if not in law, that whilst the medium on which the data are recorded belongs to the care provider, the data themselves are owned jointly by provider and patient with some elements perhaps being owned more by one than the other (eg interpretation, decisions and business records may be more the providers property; the raw data and observations may be more owned by the subject). Whilst ownership of the data may be clouded, it is clear that both patient and provider have rights of access to the data and that the record keeper has a duty of proper custodianship. It may be a condition of care purchased by a third party that certain parts of the record are made available also to the purchaser for claims management and administration. However the amount of data required for these non-clinical purposes is only a very small part of the complete record, and, after validation of the patient identity, the remainder of the claims administration can be completed separated from all patient identifiers.

As to the remainder of the data, however commercially valuable it might be potentially, it cannot ethically be used if it identifies the subject in any way without the express consent of the subject: to so do would be in breach of custom and common practice, of the ethics of health professionals, and of international information principles as set down, for example, by the OECD (1) (information may not be used for any purpose other than that for which it was given).

Whilst many elements of the individual medical record may not be of any great sensitivity, most patients will feel sensitive about some elements, and almost all individuals resent intrusions into their personal information space, some more than others. The crucial issue in any discussion of privacy and confidentiality, is that once data are known to an individual, even if that knowledge is acquired by chance or accident, they cannot be unknown: there is no way of turning back the clock to recreate the state of unawareness. The vast majority of deliberate abuses of confidentiality take place through misuse privileged access to information by those who are authorised users of the data. Access to confidential data by unauthorised persons remains a relatively uncommon occurrence in well managed systems. Hence it is important to restrict access to data by authorised users to the maximum compatible with effective working, and to manage and modify the behaviour of authorised users of confidential data (eg through adherence to a code of practice) such that they do not abuse their privilege. Of course this must be backed by measures to detect abuses, as well as by technical measures to prevent unauthorised access to data both in storage and in transit. And abuses, when detected, must be subject to appropriate penalties.

The above, then, identifies the five tools that are available to manage the security of a system, such as a wide area health network where personalised information is stored and communicated:

preventive strategies
detective strategies
behaviour management
perception management
redress and punishment for abuses.

Systems that are perceived as insufficiently secure will not be used, or will be used ineffectively. Both doctors and patients may withhold vital information from such systems, and the resultant deterioration in data quality will undermine the usefulness of the system. Ultimately it is perceptions that determine whether a system will be able to deliver to its full potential, and perceptions are based at least as much on emotions as they are on facts and reason. Management of the perceptions of data subjects and users of a system is a crucial factor in determining its acceptance, a key element of which is openness and proactive management: nothing undermines public confidence faster than being secretive or devious, or appearing to be.

New Zealand - A Case Study

The New Zealand Ministry of Health recognised the need for a national health information network to support the development of present and future health care services and their delivery. The system was designed to provide a point of connection for all those with a legitimate interest in health information (eg doctors, insurers, laboratories, registrars) for access to information resources and for exchange of health care messages. This environment was implemented during 1993.

The general schema of the system at the present time is as shown in figure 1: many additional resources and services will become available as the demand and technology makes them economically viable. Details of the basic functionality and operations are given elsewhere[2,3]. An outline of the overall arrangement of the system is shown below:

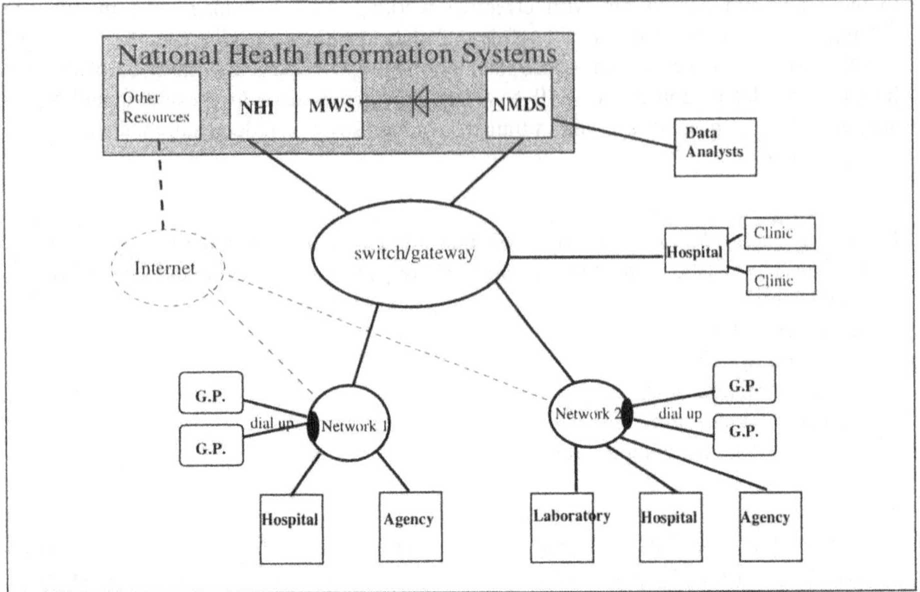

Figure 1: A schematic outline of the New Zealand National Health Information System

Below each of the elements of the National Health Information System databases which hold confidential material is briefly explained:

- **National Health Index** (NHI) database, which is a register of all users of health care services in New Zealand, and which records the unique identifier assigned to each individual for health purposes only. The NHI records the user name and aliases (alternate registrations with the same NHI number), address, date of birth, gender, NZ resident status and ethnicity, and is interactively accessible by authorised users.

- **Medical Warnings System** (MWS), which maintains a record of significant medical conditions (allergies, life threatening conditions, adverse drug reactions, life sustaining treatments etc), contact details (eg next-of-kin), donor status, as well as a synopsis of past medical care encounters. These past encounters are normally abstracted automatically from records sent to the NMDS system (see below). This system is interactively accessible to authorised care providers.

- **National Minimum Data Set** (NMDS) database, which is a record of health care events, and is gathered from all sections of the health care system (although collection of reports of primary care encounters have not yet commenced). For protection of personal privacy, this database includes no personal identifiers, other than the NHI number which is encrypted. A summary of each NMDS report is normally passed through to the MWS (see above) to appear in the past care encounters listing, but this is blocked if patient or provider have requested that it be treated in confidence (by checking a box in the submittal message). Care providers send messages to the NMDS in batch mode: access to the NMDS database is limited to a relatively small group of statisticians.

Issues of personal privacy and system security occupied a key role throughout the planning and development of this system. It was recognised from the start that this would be a crucial factor in determining its acceptability to provider and community alike.

Prevailing Legislation

New Zealand enacted a Privacy Act[4] in 1993. The Act is generic and applies to all information whether publicly or privately owned: each sector is responsible for developing a Code of Practice, which, once approved by the Privacy Commissioner, constitutes an integral element of the overall legislation. The health sector Code of Practice[5] addresses each of the 14 rules laid down in the Act, which align closely with the principles outlined by the OECD[1], and explains each rule and its objective, giving guidance and examples on how it should be interpreted and applied in the health sector. The rules relate to:

1. purposes of collections of health information - must be explicitly stated and lawful
2. sources of health information - should be from the subject unless this is impossible
3. collection of information from the subject - must be with their knowledge and understanding of the purpose of the collections, who will have access to their data and the consequences of withholding data
4. manner of collection of health information - must be carried out in appropriate surroundings, in a legal manner and without unreasonably intrusion into their private affairs
5. storage and security of health information - must be protected against loss, corruption and unauthorised access
6. access to health information - must be accessible only to authorised users and to the data subject (at nominal cost)
7. correction of health information - subjects may request corrections which must be implemented or, if refused, a note attached which must be viewed with the data indicating the requested correction
8. accuracy of health information to be checked before use - must be validated wherever possible before use
9. agency not to keep health information for longer than necessary - data can only be stored whilst the intended purpose of the collection still pertains
10. limits on the use of health information - can only be used for the stated intended purpose, unless the consent of the subject is obtained
11. limits on the disclosure of health information - can only be disclosed as has been declared in (1) above, with certain exceptions, for example court order, statutory requirement, or where there is real danger of serious damage to the subject or to a third party.
12. use of sectoral unique identifiers - a unique identifier can be used for one sector only and may not be used in connection with or linked to any other sector or purpose
13. complaints procedures - are laid down
14. requirements for privacy officers - in order to implement and monitor the regulations

Viewed from the perspective of a data subject, Rule 3 requires that the subject is made aware of the purpose(s) for which data is being collected, who will hold it, who is intended to have access to it, whether it is authorised or required by law, any consequences of not providing it, and the rights of access to and correction of it. Rule 4 requires that information is collected fairly, lawfully and without unreasonable intrusion into their personal affairs. Rule 6 entitles the subject to have access to any information stored about them and sets down time limits for reaching a decision on access (20 days), grounds for refusing and permissible charges (normally nil). Rule 7 entitles the subject to request correction of information, and to have the details of any requested correction that is refused permanently attached to the information so that it must always be read with it. Rule 10 requires that information collected for one purpose can be used only for that purpose, and Rule 11 places strict limits on disclosures of information without the subjects consent, except as required to fulfill the purpose of collection. Rule 12 permits the use of a health sector unique identifier for the purposes of providing integrated care, but precludes its use by any other agency or sector.

The privacy rules and their application are explained for both professionals and patients in a series of publications prepared by various agencies - principally the Ministry of Health, the Regional Health Authorities (public care purchasers) and the Crown Health Enterprises (public secondary care provider organisations).

User Access Agreements

Every user of the system has to apply for access rights, outlining their legitimate needs for access to the information. An appropriate level of access is determined, a userID and password issued and a legal agreement is entered into between the user and the Ministry of Health. For example access to the MWS, containing personal clinical details, is restricted to registered doctors. Before the user can connect to the systems, they must:

- make arrangements with an accredited network service for communications facilities
- fulfill requirements regarding their local systems security arrangements
- arrange for their computer system to be tested, using a predetermined routine, to ensure that it complies fully with the provisions of the relevant message standards and therefore eliminating the possibility of errors arising out of communications failures or errors.

User Identification and Audit Trails

Every transaction (simply viewing data is considered to be a transaction) on the NHI/MWS systems is logged, together with the identity of the user, to create an audit trail. Some users of the system work alone (eg GPs) and have their own userID and password, which provides them with agreed access rights. This arrangement would be too inflexible to enable large organisations, such as hospitals where staff may change frequently, to function efficiently. In these situations the chief executive of the organisation can be the authorised and responsible user, and is authorised to assign access rights to staff of that organisation provided that the security arrangements on the system are acceptable. In order to provide for the needs of the audit trail, in a transaction the client (eg hospital) system passes through to the host the identity and authentication of the client (eg userID and password) together with the identification of the user on the client system/network (eg their userID) so that the two system logs together can uniquely identify the user for every transaction. In this way a new user can be registered by the client and assigned rights to use the national systems for their work without the paperwork and inevitable time delays that would otherwise ensue.

Standards - Networking and Messaging

Messages to the NHI/MWS system are interactive and carry identifying information: these messages are encrypted using a simple but effective algorithm considered adequate to counter current threats, and are exchanged using the HL7 protocol. Messages to the NMDS carry only unique identifiers without any personal data: these are sent using EDIFACT, and at present they are not encrypted, although their encryption is under consideration.

Accreditation of public networks to carry communications to the national systems involves demonstration of appropriate technology, and entering into a contract with the Ministry regarding principally security (service availability, information privacy etc) issues. Network providers are encouraged to develop whatever value added services their customers may choose, so providing them with a further incentive to promote and enhance the system.

Discussion

This case study illustrates the use of the five tools mentioned in the introduction.

Prevention. All users can be uniquely identified, and access to personalised data is restricted to the minimum consistent with the needs of the individual user. Computer systems used in connection with the national systems are checked for compliance with requirements to ensure that errors cannot arise and that security is not compromised. All NHI/MWS communications are encrypted. NMDS records are communicated with only unique identifiers from the NHI: before storage in the database these numbers are twice encrypted and thereby effectively de-identified. Inquiries of the NMDS are monitored to ensure that numerical values in all cells are greater than 6 to further minimise the possibility of identification of individuals through serial statistical analyses of event records.

Detection. Transaction logs generate audit trails which ensure that every user can be held accountable for their actions.
Behaviour management. The provisions of the Privacy Act and Code of Practice are widely publicised and explained for health professionals. Reviews of compliance with this legislation are in the hands of the office of the Privacy Commissioner.
Perception Management. Explanatory materials for patients are widely available (eg at reception desks) and are designed to make them aware of their rights. Opportunities are taken to ensure that the mass media are fully informed and therefore able to provide positive publicity. The ownership of the national systems by the government may be seen as less than ideal, given the level of concern in the community as to whether government can be trusted with personal information: however ownership by a commercial body is seen as less desirable.
Redress and punishment for abuses. The Privacy Act provides a framework for taking action against abusers. This is supplemented by the contracts between users, network services and the national systems, which also provide for action to be taken in the case of mis-use.

From the point of view of the management of claims and contracts, the intention relating to the passing of data between the various parties is as follows. The care service provider holds a full set of data relating to personal, administrative and clinical issues. A limited set of this data is passed to the respective purchaser: the purchaser should check the identifiers only to confirm that they are responsible for purchasing care for the person concerned, and then detach those identifiers before passing the clinical and administrative data on for claims and contract management. This ensures that the full set of data is not seen by anyone. Various research and analysis programs may be active: these should have no access to identified data. Cohort and longitudinal studies can readily be carried out since events relating to the same individual will always have the same identification number (which is the double encrypted NHI number). Where research must be undertaken on identified patients, their permission must be sought through their care provider(s) to this use of their data in advance, or retrospectively. Aggregated data only is available to the funders since they have no need of identified data. There are provisions for purchasers and public health officials to re-identify the subject of data sets solely in order to ensure accountability, prevent and prosecute fraud and carry out their statutory duties.

Conclusion

Too much emphasis is often placed on the use of technology alone in maintaining the security or systems and the confidentiality of the data stored on them. Technology alone cannot solve the problem of, although it has an important role to play. More important are two crucial issues: the effective management of people to promote awareness of the issues and discourage abuses of privilege, and paying careful attention to the data sets that are passed between users to ensure that they comprise the minimum required to serve the identified purposes, and that the identifiers are separated ('de-identified' data) and/or encrypted wherever they are not absolutely essential.

The system outlined above is dynamic. Plans for major enhancements are under consideration at the present time [6], which include further provision for security, increased empowerment of individuals, and mechanisms for exchanging a wide range of clinical data between providers to improve continuity and integrity of patient care.

References

1. Guidelines on the Protection of Privacy and Trans-border flows of Personal Data Paris: OECD, 1981
2. Neame RLB and Johnston J: Developing A National Health Information Network: Insights From Experiences In New Zealand, In: Proceedings of Conference on Current Perspective in Healthcare Computing (HC94), Harrogate (Ed. B Richards), BJHC: London, 1994 503-509.
3. Johnston J and Neame RLB: A National On-line Population-based Index of Healthcare Consumers: Issues and Insights from the New Zealand Experience, Proceedings of the 12th International Congress of the European Federation for Medical Informatics (MIE 94) (Eds: P Barahona, M Veloso and J Bryant) EFMI: Lisbon 1994 320-327
4. The Privacy Act, New Zealand 1993
5. Code of Practice under the Privacy Act covering health information held by health agencies. Auckland, NZ: New Zealand Privacy Commissioner. 1994
6. Health Information Strategy for the Year 2000. Wellington, New Zealand: Ministry of Health, 1996

An Update on the BMA Security Policy

Ross Anderson

Cambridge University Computer Laboratory
Pembroke Street, Cambridge CB2 3QG
ross.anderson@cl.cam.ac.uk

Abstract. In this article, we attempt to step back from the current dispute between the BMA and the government and describe it as a whole. We give a brief account of the origins and development of the BMA security policy and guidelines. We then summarise the feedback so far, and discuss its practical implications (which were the focus of official objections). Experience of pilot projects and systems overseas shows that many of the problems can be solved fairly easily by available technology.

The policy has clarified things significantly, and we now see that the remaining 'hard' problems are unavoidably political. They pit long established patient rights and professional privileges against the NHS's Information Management and Technology Strategy, which directs healthcare computing investment away from clinical systems to build a series of databases that will make personal health information available centrally to administrators. Our investigation of this has been slowed (though not thwarted) by systematic official obstruction, which suggests that administrators are uncomfortably aware of the ethical problems.

1 Introduction

In late 1994 and early 1995, the British Medical Association (BMA) repeatedly asked officials of the UK National Health Service (NHS) about encryption of data on a new data network that was being planned. The assurances received were less than convincing. They included the claim that there was no encryption expertise in Britain, and the even more bizarre claim that encryption could not be introduced until the network was in place, as the network itself would be needed to distribute the keys [65] [66] (it was later learned that encryption proposals had been spiked at the request of the intelligence community). I was therefore contacted and asked to speak to the BMA's Information Technology Committee (as it now is) on the 8th March.

On looking at the documents that the government had supplied to the BMA on security in the proposed network [50] [51] [52] [53] [54], it was clear that something was wrong. The government assumed that the main additional threat from connecting clinical computer systems together would come from outside 'hackers' — a view common enough in the popular press but not held by people with experience of the field.

The likelihood that data will be abused depends on its value and on the number of people who have access. Connecting systems together increases both these risk factors at the same time. An example is given by personal financial information, which in many countries is no longer private: as any bank teller can access any account at most banks, an illegal data broker needs only a small number of sources to cover most of the population's finances [44] [64]. The prospect of medical records suffering a similar fate is alarming, and the controls proposed by the government would have been unable to prevent this.

The NHS argument was that for 'security' reasons, all clinical data would have to be carried on their private network that was being set up by a contractor, BT. Organisations wishing to connect to it (and all significant healthcare providers would be forced to) would have to sign a 'Code of Connection' promising not to connect their systems to any other network [54]. But however convenient the Code for BT's business at a time of rapidly growing competition and falling costs for data network services, it would provide no protection against the majority of attackers who would, we believed, come from inside the system rather than from outside.

Our concerns were first communicated to the government in detail in a letter from the BMA on the 21st March 1995. This questioned the assumptions that the NHS network could be kept separate from the Internet and that encryption was infeasible; it also pointed out inconsistencies in the NHS security policy. It received a testy response. Thus, on the 31st May, the BMA Council supported a resolution from the IT working party that the problems with the threat model, security policy and architecture would "need to be addressed as a matter of urgency by the NHS Executive or use of the NHS Wide Network would be boycotted for the transmission of identifiable patient data by doctors concerned about confidentiality".

So we prepared a detailed critique [4] of the NHS threat model, security policy and architecture and presented it to senior officials on the 8th June 1995. At that time, we fully accepted the bona fides of the NHS Executive and aimed to help them revise their security policy and architecture documents to be acceptable. In the world of security, it is common practice that one party advances a design and another tries to find holes in it. Such third party evaluation is a standard industry practice, and is mandatory in many government systems in Britain, the EU [39] and elsewhere.

2 The Gathering Storm

We were not to know it at the time, but the NHS Executive had projects underway to build systems that are in serious conflict with medical ethics as understood by both doctors [31] [32] and patients [17] [36] [59]. If security rules are adopted that enforce this traditional view, then these systems will require significant changes (which we discuss below).

So, with the benefit of hindsight, it is not at all surprising that the response we received from the NHS Executive was limited to nitpicking [47], ad hominem attacks, diversionary tactics (such as the recent report on encryption [77]) and delay.

This surpassed the script of "Yes Minister". For example, at a meeting called on the 26th June to present their response to our critique, officials claimed that we would have to wait for the NHS to settle its confidentiality policy — a document that had been stalled for some 15 years, and the most recent version of which (in August 1994 [14]) had been roundly rejected by clinical professions, patients and the Data Protection Registrar. So the Association went public with its concerns; these were summarised in an article that appeared in July [3].

By then it had become rather clear that the government was determined on a tactical rather than constructive response. Our intelligence sources reported a determination to implement the Code of Connection and deal with objectors by obfuscation, delay and diversion; the strategy was to field the network and present it as a fait accompli. Typical of the tactics used in this period was a letter in September that sought to query the minutes of the 26th June meeting and wished a further meeting in November to discuss them [48]. Also in September, a senior IMG official claimed at a conference that our criticisms had been completely misguided, as the primary purpose of the NHS network was to provide leased lines between hospitals that would cut phone bills!

In spite of these Fabian tactics, the foundations of the government's position were removed one by one. The erroneous initial assumption — that the main additional threat from networking would come from outsiders — was repudiated in a report commissioned by NHS managers from the government's own expert body, the CCTA [55]; the four level 'classification' of data that formed the intellectual core of their security policy and justified their architecture was next to go [67]; yet officials stuck adamantly to their 'Code of Connection'. In vain we pointed out the practical problems that would arise — Addenbrookes' Hospital, for example, shares its network infrastructure with Cambridge University. These objections were ignored.

More senior officials became involved, and their tactics became steadily more reckless. A very senior medical officer wrote in August that the government would press ahead with its Code of Connection and hoped that the BMA objections could be dealt with later [75]; when we objected to the use of the network for clinical information, he claimed that Item-of-Service claims were not personal health information and that contract minimum data sets were 'of course coded' [76]. For the benefit of readers not familiar with NHS systems, a typical Item-of-Service claim is for the supply by a general practitioner of contraceptive care, and that a typical contract minimum data set is for an episode of hospital treatment. I was personally lost for words that one of the government's most eminent doctors could hold unworthy of protection the identities of under-age girls taking the pill or obtaining pregnancy terminations in NHS hospitals.

On the 8th December 1995, the Code of Connection was issued, despite senior officials having given assurances to the BMA on the same day that this would not happen [27]; it was promptly denounced by the Association [28]. The Code, together with supporting documents such as the IS Security Reference Manual [56], continued to use the security assumptions and arguments that had already been discredited by the government's own experts.

We pointed this out and on the 13th December a senior official wrote to the Association:

> You have included references to IMG project documents. These are project working papers provided to project members ... you will see that they are classified "Restricted: Management" ... please therefore delete the references [67].

No assurances of confidentiality had been sought by the government, or given by the Association, when these documents were originally supplied.

3 The Policy is Commissioned

By September 1995, the BMA had become convinced that the NHS Executive either would not or could not draw up an acceptable security policy, and so on the 7th October the BMA Council asked me to do this. My goal was not to rewrite the traditional ethics of the profession, but to translate them into a concise set of rules that would provide a clear and unambiguous basis of communication between patients, clinicians and policymakers on the one hand, and computer system builders on the other.

There already existed two well understood security policy models to provide some inspiration. The first is the Bell-LaPadula policy, used by the world's armed forces, under which an official cleared to 'secret' should be able to see documents classified 'secret' and below, but nothing at 'top secret' or above. In other words, information only flows upwards, and never downwards, through a hierarchy of security levels [9]. The second is the Clark-Wilson policy that was developed to formalise good practice in banking and bookkeeping systems, and which lays down a number of rules to enforce controls such as dual control and audit [19]. But neither of these would do for clinical information, the basic principle of which is expressed by the General Medical Council [31] as:

> Patients have a right to expect that you will not pass on any personal information which you learn in the course of your professional duties, unless they agree.

Thus our goal is patient control of data access, rather than an access hierarchy that reflects an organisational command structure. It is privacy, that empowers the patient, rather than confidentiality, that empowers the organisation. This distinction is already familiar to medical ethicists: in English law, the privacy of medical records is founded on the rights of the patient while the confidentiality of social work records is based on the rights of the local authority that employs the social worker [24]. However, it was less familiar in the computer security world, as previous security models (including both Bell-LaPadula and Clark-Wilson) had been driven by organisational rather than privacy concerns.

So how could privacy — the principle of patient control — be encapsulated in a compact set of rules that would be easily understood by patients and clinicians, but sufficiently precise for system builders?

The BMA also commissioned guidelines. The idea was that the policy would be normative — it would state where we should be in a few years' time — while the guidelines would tell the working doctor how to protect her patients (and herself) from the immediate threats. One might think of the policy as the long-term treatment plan, and the guidelines as a bandage to stop the bleeding.

Developing the policy was a fascinating experience. The main primary sources used to elucidate the GMC position were the books by Somerville on medical ethics [72], and by Darley, Griew, McLoughlin and Williams on clinical confidentiality [24]. These provided the background material on what problems arise in practice, and how the clinical professions expect them to be dealt with. The pioneering study of electronic patient records by Griew and Currell [30] was also useful; it showed how complex it is to build a policy model for a record containing components to which different combinations of clinicians would have access, and motivated the search for a simpler framework.

The key idea was to assume that each record would have a unique access policy. That is, we would treat a lifetime's medical history as an accumulation of records, each of which was completely accessible to a the same set of users. Thus the general record might be available to everyone in a practice or care team, while a note on a treatment for depression might be open only to the doctor who treated it (and to the patient). This greatly simplifies things, and has the virtue of reflecting actual clinical practice.

By early November 1995, a first draft of the policy was circulated, and was significantly refined by a number of discussions. Among the most helpful were presentations to the BMA's IT and Ethics committees; we also shared the early drafts with software suppliers so that any practical objections could be raised, and with the NHS Executive, whose contribution at the time was negligible. These meetings took place during November and December 1995.

The final versions of the policy and guidelines were written over the New Year holiday and shipped in early January 1996 [5] [6]. The core of the policy is contained in nine principles, which are appended. A period of public consultation ensued, of which this workshop is the logical culmination.

4 Post Publication Feedback

The feedback on the security policy, from both institutions and individuals, has been roughly of three kinds. Firstly, the majority of responses have been strongly supportive (e.g., [26]). A common comment has been that the work brings clarity to a subject that many had for years found to be confusing, and that while its principles may not all be achievable at once (or even at all in some legacy systems), it shows where we should be going. At least one medical school has dicussed incorporating the policy into its curriculum.

The second kind of response has come from officialdom and its sympathisers, who emphasise 'practical' objections to the policy. This became amusingly clear at a meeting with officials on the 6th February at which a senior official claimed that the principles would be impractical, as the notification requirements would be too onerous. We informed him that we would be resolving this question by conducting a trial at a number of general practices. He then said that although the principles might work in general practice, they might be impractical in a hospital setting. A clinician present asked whether he was suggesting a trial in the context of GP-hospital links and he replied that that would be an adequate trial. We promptly agreed and minuted the agreement. In a later letter, he complained that this was still not wide enough to test the principles' practicality [68].

The rest of the criticisms — the interesting and useful kind — are made up of a large number of observations by various parties, but with a number of recurring themes.

1. A number of clinicians have argued that integrated hospital systems can bring important safety benefits; they might help prevent the tragedies that can happen when records go astray (as many paper records do [1] [2]). The point is also made that at some hospitals, as many as 70% of admissions are accident and emergency, so there is little scope for compartmentation between clinical departments [63]. When one asks advocates of integrated hospital systems how to control the aggregation threat that arises when many hospital staff can see data on many patients, and which will become much worse if hospitals are connected together into a network, the suggestions include:
   - forego NHS networking as insufficiently important;
   - allow only a small number of trusted staff to copy records from one hospital to another, and audit them closely;
   - remove general access to records of patients who are not currently receiving treatment. A typical acute hospital might have files on a million people, but only a few percent might be active (as in- or out-patients) at any one time. Only a small number of trusted library and admissions staff would have the ability to restore a record to 'active' status;
   - our suggestion was to use a technology such as active badges [73] to track hospital staff, and prevent (or investigate) accesses to the records of patients in other departments or wards. It turns out that a similar system is used in some US hospitals but based on departmental groups of terminals. Staff who access another department's records face questioning and possible disciplinary action [23];
   - educate the public to change their expectations of medical privacy.

   In any case, the practicality of securing hospital information systems is an open question, with some contributors foreseeing serious problems [63] and others not [35]. Resolving this will be an empirical matter, and may involve some exceptions to the policy — an issue which we will discuss further below.
2. One of the most trenchant criticisms came from a senior member of the computer security community, Gus Simmons (who was for many years the senior scientist at Sandia National Laboratories, whose responsibilities include the security of the US nuclear arsenal). He argued that it is not adequate to secure an electronic system to the same level as the paper system it replaces, as critical social controls are removed.

With a paper records system, an attacker can always grab a file from someone else's office, but this activity is counter to social taboos, and is fraught with risk that the occupant might return unexpectedly. But when records are placed on a computer, anyone who can get access through his terminal will not appear to a passer-by be doing anything wrong. Thus he may feel that he is committing at most a very minor misdemeanour. So electronic record keeping systems should have very strong auditing and intrusion detection systems; a deterrent that must be publicised and credible [71].

3. As an intrusion detection mechanism, Simmons suggested that whenever anyone looked at a patient's record but did not bill the patient for her time, then it should be investigated as a prima facie abuse. This would harmonise the patient's interest in privacy and the hospital management's interest in maximising its revenue.
4. Similar ideas were suggested independently by Ulrich Kohl [43]. His development is somewhat more general and shows that context-based access controls can be implemented with with quite general parameters.
5. On the other extreme, the policy has been criticised for not emphasising that computerised medical records have the capability to be much more secure than paper records [63]. We have never disputed this as a possibility — but have still to see a really secure electronic medical record system fielded.
6. A number of contributors worried about the extent to which access control lists would have to be micromanaged, and whether this would turn out to be a serious burden given the large number of record fragments that can pertain to one individual [62]. In fact, given the signal-to-noise problems, might it not turn out to be unfeasible?

   Our view was that the great majority of individuals can be dealt with using a default access control list, containing a group such as 'all GPs working in the practice', and that only a small number of highly sensitive records would require exceptional treatment with an access control list containing only the treating doctor and the patient himself. Nonetheless this was felt to be an extremely important question, and in consequence was one of the points investigated in a trial of the principles carried out in a number of general practices. Some early results are described in the paper by Alan Hassey and Mike Wells [36].
7. A number of contributors objected to the restrictions on aggregating patient data. A typical comment was "There is no doubt that general aggregated data, such as immunisation uptake, has been beneficial to the common good ... system linkage or networking has, I would suggest, been poorly planned and perhaps somewhat hurried ... however I do feel that it is inevitable and that the benefits will ultimately outweight the perceived pitfalls" [60]. Several groups opined that with de-identified data it might be extremely difficult to obtain information such as analysis of readmissions to hospitals [22] [70]. This is a very important point, and one on which US contributors also had much to say; we will deal with it fully in a later section.
8. Tom Rindfleisch made the point, with which we fully agree, that informed

consent should not be sought at the stressful point of critical need, but in advance, like a living will [62]. A related point is made by the German information security agency: that for consent to be meaningful, systems must be designed so that people who refuse to use part or all of them, or to grant some information access, do not lose their right to care as a result [10]. The German case referred to a health smartcard; it is unclear what would happen if someone needing hospital treatment in the UK refused permission for their personal health information to be entered on the Clearing system, and discussions with officials have elicited only the vague suggestion that perhaps the hospital would simply foot the bill for treatment itself "as a one-off".

9. Some members of the computer security community objected to principle 9 (the Trusted Computing Base), on the grounds that it is a part of the security engineer's basic intellectual environment. However, the BMA policy talks to clinicians as well as technicians, so we feel it is appropriate. No matter how the document is written there will be parts that some section of the audience feels to be superfluous.
10. Some writers preferred 'fuzzier' statements of the security policy goals and want it to be more 'patient centred' [61]. We remain unmoved. A security policy is like a scalpel: it must be clean and sharp rather than warm and furry. As for the buzzword 'patient centred', systems so described often seem to be a cover for transferring the primary record from the GP to a health authority, a hospital or an insurance company. We are satisfied to have upheld the principle of patient control.
11. A number of computer companies complained that the security functionality required was so different from that offered by their current products that expensive redevelopment would be necessary [11]; while the Association of the British Pharmaceutical Industry asked for some of the principles to be made less 'draconian' [74].
12. We received quite a lot of input on practical solutions used elsewhere, e.g. German cancer registries [12], the New Zealand registry system [58], and similar registries registries implemented in Denmark [45] and proposed in Norway [13]. The point was also made — from experience with HIV programmes in the USA — that apart from neonates, the date of birth is clinically irrelevant and should be suppressed in clinical systems, thereby reducing the likelihood of harmful linkages being constructed with other systems at some later date [15].

We noted above that some exceptions to the policy may have to be made, e.g. for accident and emergency staff. This does not of course invalidate the policy. Even policies such as Bell LaPadula and Clark-Wilson fail to cover their application areas completely. In a bank, for example, there are typically about twenty roles which cannot realistically be subjected to dual control, such as the chief executive, the chief systems programmer, the computer security manager and the chief dealer. Such people simply have to be trusted, despite the fact that the trust occasionally turns out to be misplaced.

This is well understood in the security comunity. The security policy sets a yardstick; system builders get as close to it as they economically can; the shortcomings are examined during the evaluation process; and so when the system is presented by the contractor to the customer, he can make an informed decision on whether to accept the residual risk or send the system back for redevelopment. The policy does not eliminate residual risk, but rather quantifies it and enables a prudent judgment to be made about it.

That kind of benefit should materialise once people start using the policy to build systems. Meantime the main benefit is clarity. The policy has enabled us to work through the logical consequences of the GMC's ethical principle — that patients should have control over access — in much greater detail than ever before, and apply it as a test to many fielded and proposed systems.

Previously, discussions had tended to set a rather poorly defined 'patient confidentiality' against an equally poorly defined 'public interest' that was often described vaguely in terms of research benefits but was all too often a front for attempts to increase official power and control. However the policy, and its followup in the GP pilot, brought us to identify the tension between privacy and safety as the best way to express the trade-offs from the patient's point of view.

Leaflets distributed as part of the GP pilot reflect this, and the GP pilot also enabled us to identify the flows of information from general practice to health authorities, for such purposes as item-of-service claims and cervical screening, as one of the few problems with implementing the policy and guidelines in general practice [42] [36].

It also brought to our attention that there are potentially major problems with de-identification of the data in statistical databases. However, before we explore this, it is appropriate to mention the feedback received from conferences in the USA.

5 A Lesson from America

A version of the BMA security policy was accepted for presentation at the IEEE Symposium on Security and Privacy at Oakland, which is the premier conference on computer security, and we submitted a condensed version that incorporated much of the early feedback [8]. After the paper was presented (on the 7th May), there was a panel discussion at which an academic, a doctor and a representative of the healthcare computing industry presented their views of the policy. Then, on the 10th May, the policy was presented again at a workshop in Washington at which doctors, lawyers, rights activists and congressional staffers discussed the issues from a US viewpoint.

The main lesson learned from this trip was that the real privacy problem in the USA comes from the claims databases operated by the insurance companies that pay for most US healthcare. These databases are coming to replace the casenotes in the doctor's office as the primary record for many Americans; the convenience of having a lifetime's record in one place outweighs the fact that these records were not generally designed for clinical use.

The sidelines the security debate. US hospital computer systems have much greater variety than their UK counterparts, and their level degree of security also varies widely. But there is a feeling that, since patient records can be obtained by almost anyone from the insurance industry, why should more money be invested in making hospital systems any better?

One of the Oakland speakers revealed that his company sees the seven million records kept by its health systems division as a major business asset, and would strongly resist any attempt by legislators or others to restrict the ways in which this could be used to produce revenue. As we noted in the policy, this business structure has led to practices that would be considered highly abusive in the UK. For example, forty percent of insurers disclose personal health information to lenders, employers or marketers without customer permission [18]; over half of America's largest 500 companies admitted using health records in personnel decisions [16]; and US firms are regularly taken over for the value of the medical records under their control. Indeed, most Americans are coming to feel that these practices are worrying, and a quarter have personal experience of abuse [33].

This has led to a number of bills being introduced or proposed at both state and federal level, and is the subject of papers elsewhere in this volume. Here we will remark that aggregated records make a tempting target. For example, at the Washington meeting a district attorney discussed his use of medical records in criminal investigations. He saw nothing remiss in issuing a subpoena for insurance company files that he thought might be helpful — and insurance files (being considered financial rather than health records) enjoyed no special privilege.

Another serious aspect of claims-based longitudinal records is that they are not accurate. It is common to 'inflate' diagnoses so as to be able to claim higher fees, so that, for example, non-specific chest pain will be recorded as ischaemic heart disease. This might be qualified as a tentative diagnosis in the clinical notes, but as the 'unified computer record' supersedes this, the false diagnosis may prevail. It was mentioned that some 20% of alleged clinical facts in the computer record were wrong; if this is even the right order of magnitude, then the risks to health are significant.

The social effects of insurance-driven data aggregation are also becoming understood. At the Washington meeting, a primary care physician told us that over the last twenty years, US patients have moved from complete trust in their family doctor to a much more guarded relationship, in which patients suppress facts that are potentially embarrassing or harmful. The risks of this should also be clear.

6 Could it Happen Here?

The standard response of NHS officials on being told of information abuses in the United States is 'it couldn't happen here'. Yet the US trip focussed our attention on the threat from the construction of large databases of personal health information. There had already been signs that all was not well.

An internal presentation by the NHS Executive to the effect that there should be a unified electronic patient record, shared by everyone in the NHS, had already caused concern — to the extent that we had confronted senior officials on the 31st January and asked whether the real goal of the IM&T strategy was to construct a series of centralised databases, each covering a different aspect of health care but which would together contain essentially all personal health information on every NHS patient — in effect, nationalising the country's medical records using contract data as the Trojan Horse for the project.

This was stoutly denied. Officials categorically assured us that the abstracts of the contract data that were kept centrally were not only de-identified, but also unlinkable — separate episodes concerning the same patient could not be correlated. This was claimed to be a property of the HES data formats. We accepted these assurances and asked for a copy of the HES data specifications; we were promised a copy (which never turned up). Incidentally, the claim that central databases contain only episode data is still being repeated by senior officials [49].

The next stimulus came in February 1996 from an HIV data collection project. This was presented as an attempt to improve planning for HIV sufferers, who at present can self-refer to any hospital in the UK rather than having to go through their GP. As a result, officials suspected that the 18,000 registered sufferers represented only about 12,000 actual patients, and wanted to know if budgets could be cut. A form was sent out to all GPs and genitourinary clinics demanding details of all patients receiving treatment [46]. In addition to clinical information, this demanded that the patient be identified by date of birth, post-code and the 'Soundex' code of their surname[1]; the instructions for generating a Soundex code have the curious final line 'Note: it is very helpful if you can give the initial of the first name as well'.

This information was being chased up, and handled, by employees of district health authorities, rather than being sent directly to the Public Health Laboratory Service. The development of regional databases is also mentioned in the protocol, but without detail. When these concerns were made public, a consultant epidemiologist at the laboratory claimed that "Somebody who does not know what the Soundex code is would have no possibility of guessing the identity" [37] — hardly reassuring given that the Soundex system is public and that the patient's name and data of birth are present on the form!

Meanwhile, it was pointed out that HIV status was already encoded in the contract minimum data set, as were codes for other sexually transmitted diseases, abortions and fertility treatment [34].

The next stimulus was in March 1996 when a study of the NHS Executive's IM&T strategy commissioned by the BMA's IT Committee reported that

> The changes to the flows and management of health information will, when completed, represent the most fundamental and challenging changes to the practice of medicine ever [57].

[1] essentially, this means the initial letter and the next three consonants

7 Linkable After All!

Given this background, the US experience caused us to stop and reexamine the overall pattern, which entailed looking at the ultimate repository and beneficiaries of the large quantities of information that the Information Management and Technology Strategy sets out to gather. We had still not received the HES data definitions that the government had promised in January, so these were now obtained otherwise.

This led to the shocking discovery that the categorical assurances which we had received about the HES data were completely false. The records in this database contain the full postcode, date of birth and sex [25]. So with a few exceptions (such as twins living together, and students in colleges) the patients are easily identifiable and the episodes are linkable. In fact, it is unclear what their value would have been otherwise, as one of their avowed functions is to assess hospital readmission rates.

This contributed to an impression that the Department of Health has for some time worked to create a set of central databases with details of every episode of care in the country. If this is the case, then no doubt knowing that it would be controversial, they have tried to do it by stealth.

This impression is not dispelled by ministerial assurances. An MP had set down the following parliamentary question about the Clearing service, the central system for settling health care payments between purchasers and providers, and which also skims off the HES data for central government [21]:

> To ask the Secretary of State for Health, ... on what basis (contractor's) employees or managers will have access to personal data?

The government replied [38]:

> Their managers and employees are contractually bound to maintain the confidentiality of data passing through the Clearing Service, and will have no access to it.

This is intrinsically implausible to a computer security person (surely the system administrators will have access?), and when we obtained a copy of the Clearing system documentation we found that according to its security policy, staff with 'a direct operational functional requirement' would have access to personal health information, while access to information that had been 'de-identified' (i.e., with the name and address removed but with the postcode and date of birth still presumably present "shall be available to all Users for healthcare business purposes, subject to receipt by the Contractor in writing of rules imposed by the Data Protection Registry".

So it appears that our initial fears were well founded. In addition to the Clearing and HES systems mentioned above, there are databases in existence for prescriptions and planned for community care and data collected from general practice. Meanwhile, the government states that matching of official data will be allowed by officials investigating welfare fraud. Is it reasonable to hope that access will be denied to police, customs, tax officials, and indeed every official who can plead a 'need to know'?

8 The Way Forward

Even under the charitable explanation — that the government's actions are the result of blunder rather than malice — we face the unpleasant fact that the databases that are to support research and business information have been made identifiable by using, as the primary key, the combination of date of birth and postcode.

Quite apart from the privacy issue, this will cause both safety and reliability problems. Firstly, although most of the population can be uniquely identified in this way, a minority cannot — twins living at the same address, for example, and students in halls of residence (for whom the capture-recapture problem in probability theory ensures that if over 23 people of the same age are living at the same address, then at least two of them are likely to share the same date of birth). Thus, if in the absence of a paper record, an accident and emergency team digs out a HES record and acts on the information it contains, then there is a small but significant probability that they will be using the wrong person's data.

Another problem is that the linkage of records will be broken when patients move. This will distort hospital readmission statistics, as it can be assumed that changes of address will be correlated with illness (assuming illness to be correlated with unemployment, divorce and homelessness).

We would therefore recommend that, as a matter of urgency, the National Health Service — together with all its information systems contractors — cease and desist from using (date of birth, postcode) as a primary database key.

Instead, the techniques developed in Denmark and Germany should be used. Each healthcare provider submitting data centrally should use a pseudonym, whose linkage to the patient is unknown to outsiders. For example, one might pass the name and date of birth through a hash function such as SHA1 [69], together with a key unique to the provider, and take as many bits of the result as necessary to fill the fields in question. If the use of techniques that smack of cryptography is to be forbidden, then one can simply generate the pseudonyms at random (and take care to protect the file that links them to patient identities).

Either way, the use of systematic pseudonyms would lessen the risk of the wrong record being used, and also reduce the loss of information linkage — many address changes are local, and these patients remain with the same provider even when their postcode changes. It would also bring these systems into line with the established RCGP/GMSC guidance:

> no patient should be identifiable, other than to the general practitioner, from any data sent to an external organisation without the informed consent of the patient [40]

Such simple measures will not completely solve the problem, as people with access to the databases might infer a patient's identity from knowledge of part of their clinical history — as we pointed out in the policy. However it would eliminate the most serious problem and build a foundation on which further inference controls could be constructed (see, e.g., [29]).

It will also not tackle the problem that once large central databases exist, then there will be pressure for researchers to use these for reasons of economy. Official control of these databases then might have a negative effect on paradigm-breaking research. How readily would the establishment grant access to future scientists making unconventional claims, such as a link between Helicobacter Pylori and ulcers, or between Chlamydia and coronary heart disease?

9 Conclusions

The Secretary of State for Health is reacting to the success of the BMA's campaign against the NHS wide network by focussing health IT spending on precisely the objectionable components of the IM&T strategy (the NHS wide network, the new NHS number, the NHS wide Clearing service) at the expense of clinical systems [20]. This is strange for a conservative minister presumably alert to the dangers of centralisation and aware that the market in health systems is perfectly capably of matching willing buyers with willing sellers without the need for a central civil service department to set up national monopolies in service sectors which already have competitive provision.

We have advanced a possible explanation for the urgency. The government is building a series of linkable databases — Clearing, HES, PPA, registers for HIV, diabetes and other expensive diseases, and future databases covering primary and community care. These will eventually aggregate under central control all personal health information of significance. Although they are represented as being 'anonymised', they are nothing of the kind. The project may be justified internally as 'creating an electronic patient record shared throughout the NHS', but externally the picture is different. Officials are so sensitive about it that they have systematically obfuscated and delayed; it has taken over a year for us to dig down through successive layers to the heart of the problem.

But it is not necessary for these databases to contain identifiable information. In fact, as we have shown, replacing the current primary database key of postcode and date of birth with a one-way hash function of name and date of birth would bring tangible safety and accuracy gains.

If the database building project proceeds without controls of this kind, it can only be construed as a political attempt to centralise personal health information for state purposes. If that comes to pass, we may expect that health privacy in Britain will go the way of America. The papers in this volume by observers of the American scene give us some idea what to expect then.

Appendix — the BMA Security Policy Principles

Principle 1: Access control Each identifiable clinical record shall be marked with an access control list naming the people or groups of people who may read it and append data to it. The system shall prevent anyone not on the access control list from accessing the record in any way

Principle 2: Record opening A clinician may open a record with herself and the patient on the access control list. Where a patient has been referred, she may open a record with herself, the patient and the referring clinician(s) on the access control list

Principle 3: Control One of the clinicians on the access control list must be marked as being responsible. Only she may alter the access control list, and she may only add other health care professionals to it

Principle 4: Consent and notification The responsible clinician must notify the patient of the names on his record's access control list when it is opened, of all subsequent additions, and whenever responsibility is transferred. His consent must also be obtained, except in emergency or in the case of statutory exemptions

Principle 5: Persistence No-one shall have the ability to delete clinical information until the appropriate time period has expired

Principle 6: Attribution All accesses to clinical records shall be marked on the record with the subject's name, as well as the date and time. An audit trail must also be kept of all deletions

Principle 7: Information flow Information derived from record A may be appended to record B if and only if B's access control list is contained in A's

Principle 8: Aggregation control There shall be effective measures to prevent the aggregation of personal health information. In particular, patients must receive special notification if any person whom it is proposed to add to their access control list already has access to personal health information on a large number of people

Principle 9: Trusted Computing Base Computer systems that handle personal health information shall have a subsystem that enforces the above principles in an effective way. Its effectiveness shall be subject to evaluation by independent experts.

References

1. *'Setting the Records Straight — A Study of Hospital Medical Records'*, Audit Commission,, June 1995
2. *'For Your Information — A Study of Information Management and Systems in the Acute Hospital'*, Audit Commission,, July 1995
3. "NHS wide networking and patient confidentiality", RJ Anderson, in *British Medical Journal* v 310 no 6996 (1 July 1996) pp 5–6
4. *'NHS Network Security'*, RJ Anderson, 30th May 1995
5. *'Security in Clinical Information Systems'*, RJ Anderson, published by the British Medical Association, January 1996; also available from `http://www.cl.cam.ac.uk/users/rja14/#Med`
6. "Clinical system security: interim guidelines", RJ Anderson, in *British Medical Journal* v 312 no 7023 (13 Jan 1996) pp 109–111

7. "Patient Confidentiality — At Risk from NHS Wide Networking", RJ Anderson, *to appear in Proceedings of Healthcare 96, March 96*
8. "A Security Policy Model for Clinical Information Systems", in *Proceedings of the 1996 IEEE Symposium on Security and Privacy* pp 30–43
9. DE Bell, LJ LaPadula, *'Secure Computer Systems: Mathematical Foundations'*, Mitre Corporation report ESD-TR-73-278
10. *'Chipkarten im Gesundheitswesen'*, Bundesamt für Sicherheit in der Informationstechnik, Bundesanzeiger 4 May 1995
11. *Submission from HBO & Company*, J Baker
12. B Blobel, *this volume*
13. *'Pseudonymous Medical Registries'*, E Boe, Norwegian Official Report 1993:22
14. *'Draft guidance for the NHS on the confidentiality, use and disclosure of personal health information'*, N Boyd, DoH, 10 August 1994
15. V Brannigan, *personal communication*
16. "Is your health history anyone's business?" McCall's Magazine 4/95 p 54, reported by M Bruce on Usenet newsgroup comp.society.privacy, 22 Mar 1995
17. "Confidentiality of medical records: the patient's perspective", D Carman, N Britten, British Journal of General Practice v 45 (September 95) pp 485–488
18. "Who's reading your medical records?" *Consumer Reports*, Oct 94 pp 628–632
19. "A Comparison of Commercial and Military Computer Security Policies", D Clark, D Wilson, in *Proceedings of the 1987 IEEE Symposium on Security and Privacy* pp 184–194
20. "Dorrell urges refocus over NHS technology", in *Computer Weekly* (30/5/96)
21. Parliamentary question, H Cohen, 3/4/96
22. *'Security in Clinical Information Systems'*, submission from J Crown, President, Faculty of Public Health Medicine, to BMA, 29/2/96
23. R Cushman, *this volume*
24. *'How to Keep a Clinical Confidence'*, B Darley, A Griew, K McLoughlin, J Williams, HMSO 1994
25. *NHS Data Manual, Technical Modules Volume 1 and 2*, 1996
26. *Submission from the Society of Occupational Medicine*, D Dean, 12/4/96
27. "New Guidance on Computer Security Issued", *DoH press release*, 8/12/96
28. "BMA warns doctors about government guidance on computer security", *BMA press release*, 11/12/96
29. *'Cryptography and Data Security'*, DER Denning, Addison-Wesley 1982
30. *'A Strategy for Security of the Electronic Patient Record'*, A Griew, R Currell, IHI, University of Wales, Aberystwyth, 14/3/95
31. *'Good Medical Practice'*, General Medical Council
32. *'Confidentiality'*, General Medical Council
33. "Privacy and Security of Personal Information in a New Health Care System", LO Gostin, J Turek-Brezina, M Powers et al., in *Journal of the American Medical Association* v 20 (24/11/93) pp 2487–2493
34. "Contract minimum dataset includes confidential data", in *British Medical Journal* v 312 (20/1/96) p 185
35. *(HISS presentation to BMA IT Committee, 24/4/96)*
36. A Hassey, M Wells, *this volume*
37. "HIV code prompts debate on privacy", P Hagan, in *Hospital Doctor* (29/2/96) pp 16
38. Parliamentary reply, J Horam, 16/4/96

39. *'Information Technology Security Evaluation Criteria'*, EU document COM(90) 314 (6/91)
40. "GMSC and RCGP guidelines for the extraction and use of data from general practitioner computer systems by organisations external to the practice", Appendix III in *'Committee on Standards of Data Extraction from General Practice Guidelines'* Joint Computer Group of the GMSC and the RCGP, 1988
41. "Nurse Jailed for Hacking into Computerised Prescription System", in *British Journal of Healthcare Computing and Information Management* v 1 (94) p 7
42. S Jenkins, *this volume*
43. U Kohl, *this volume*
44. "Your Secrets for Sale", N Luck, J Burns, *The Daily Express*, 16/2/94 pp 32–33
45. *Private conversation with Peter Landrock*
46. " 'Soundex' codes of surnames provide confidentiality and accuracy in a national HIV database", JY Mortimer, JA Salathiel, Communicable Disease Report v 5 no 12 (10 Nov 1995) pp R183–R186
47. Senior IMG official, letter to BMA, 22/6/95
48. Senior IMG official, letter to BMA, 7/9/95
49. Senior IMG official, talk on Radio Northampton, 11.10, 12/6/96
50. *'Information Systems Security: Top level policy for the NHS'*, IMG document 2009 (b)
51. *'NWN Threats and Vulnerabilities'*, 5 April 1995, IMG document NWNS/T1.22
52. *'NHS-wide networking: data security policy'*, IMG document NWNS/T3.3
53. *'NHS wide networking security architecture'*, 3 April 1995, IMG document NWNS/T1.21
54. *Security Guide for IM&T Specialists'*, 3 April 1995, IMG document NWNS/T5.11
55. *'NHS/CCTA Internet Security Report'* version 1.3
56. *'NHS IS Reference Manual'*, December 1995
57. *'A Members' Guide to the Intended Goals and Purposes of the IM&T Strategy'* R Neame, 3/3/96
58. R Neame, *this volume*
59. "GP Practice computer security survey", RA Pitchford, S Kay, Journal of Informatics in Primary Care (September 95) pp 6–12
60. *letter from DR Price to BMA, 28/5/96*
61. M Rigby, *this volume*
62. *Presentation to IEEE Symposium on Security and Privacy 96*, T Rindfleisch, 7/5/96
63. R Roberts et al, *this volume*
64. "For Sale: your secret medical records for £150", L Rogers, D Leppard, *Sunday Times* 26/11/95 pp 1–2
65. Senior NHS Executive official, letter to BMA, 20/12/94
66. Senior NHS Executive official, letter to BMA, 15/2/95
67. Senior NHS Executive official, letter to BMA, 13/12/96
68. Senior NHS Executive official, letter to BMA, 12/2/96
69. *'Applied Cryptography'*, B Schneier, second edition, Wiley 1995
70. *Response on behalf of Conference Information Group*, Prof. M Severs
71. GJ Simmons, *personal communication, 1996*
72. *'Medical Ethics Today — Its Practice and Philosophy'*, A Sommerville, BMA 1993
73. "The Active Badge Location System", R Want, A Hopper, V Falcao, J Gibbons, in *ACM Transactions on Information Systems* v 10 no 1 (January 1992) pp 91–102
74. *Submission on behalf of the ABPI*, F Wells

75. Senior NHS medical officer, letter to BMA, 15/8/95
76. Senior NHS medical officer, letter to BMA, 17/11/95
77. *'The use of encryption and related services with the NHSnet'*, prepared by Zergo Ltd for NHS Executive; document NHSE IMG E5254

Index

Springer and the environment